Longevity Training-Book 4-Your Spiritual Connection

Copyright Page

The book is copyrighted for 2018

Longevity Training-Book 4-Your Spiritual Connection

By Martin K. Ettington

All Rights Reserved USA 2018

ISBN: 9781791664275

Printed in the United States of America

Longevity Training-Book 4-Your Spiritual Connection

Longevity Training-Book 4-Your Spiritual Connection

This book is a transcription and reproduction of the training course materials from Course #4 "Your Spiritual Connection"

In this course we spent a lot of time on your Spiritual Connection. No matter what religion or belief system you have, it's important to have some type of connection to God.

This connection is really to your inner spirit which lives outside of time and space.

There are various ways to connect to your spirit through prayer, meditation, and communing with nature. What is important is that you do something.

This connection is the most important thing you can do to build your long term health and happiness.

Longevity Training-Book 4-Your Spiritual Connection

Longevity Training-Book 4-Your Spiritual Connection

Other books by Martin K. Ettington

Spiritual and Metaphysics Books:
Prophecy: A History and How to Guide
God Like Powers and Abilities
Enlightenment for Newbies
Removing Illusions to Find True
    Happiness
Using the Scientific Method to Study
    the Paranormal
A Compendium of Metaphysics and
    How to Guides (Six books
    together in one volume)
Love from the Heart
The Enlightenment Experience
Learn Your Soul's Purpose
Pursuing Enlightenment
A Modern Man's Search for Truth
Use Intuition and Prophecy to Improve
    Your Life
The Handbook of Spiritual and Energy
    Healing

Longevity & Immortality:
Physical Immortality: A History and
    How to Guide
The Commentaries of Living Immortals
Records of Extremely Long Lived
    Persons
Enlightenment and Immortality
Longevity Improvements from Science
The 10 Principles of Personal
    Longevity
Telomeres & Longevity
The Diets and Lifestyles of the Worlds
    Oldest Peoples
The Longevity Six Books Bundle

Science Fiction:
Out of This Universe
Personal Freedom-Parts 1 & 2
The Psychic Soldier Series:
    Book 1-Himalayan Journey
    Book 2-A Soldier is Born
    Book 3-Fighting For Right
    Book 4-Earth Protector
The Immortality Sci Fi Bundle

The God Like Powers Series:
Human Invisibility
Invulnerability and Shielding
Teleportation
Psychokinesis
Our Energy Body, Auras, and
Thoughtforms

The God Like Powers Series—
    Volume 1 Compilation
The Yoga Discovery Series:
Yoga-An Ancient Art Form
Hatha Yoga-Helping you Live Better
Raja Yoga-Through the Ages
The Yoga Discovery Package

Business & Coaching Books:
Creating, Paublishing, & Marketing
    Practitioner Ebooks
Building a Successful Longevity
    Coaching Business
Why Become a Coach?
The Professional Coaching Success
Trilogy
2020-Make Money Writing and Selling
    Books
The 2020 Handbook of High Paying
    Work Without a College Degree

Science, Technology, and Misc.
Future Predictions By and Engineer &
    Seer
The Unusual Science & Technology
    Bundle
The Real Atlantis-In the Eye of the
    Sahara
Are Cryptozoological Animals Real or
    Imaginary?
Real Time Travel Stories From a
    Psychic Engineer
Removing Limits On Our
    Consciousness-And
    Thinking Outside the Box
33 Incredible True Survival Stories
How to Survive Anything: From the
    Wilderness to Man Made
    Disasters
All About Mars Journeys and
    Settlement
Mining the Asteroid Belt

Ancient History
The Real Atlantis-In the Eye of the
Sahara
Ancient & Prehistoric Civilizations
Ancient & Prehistoric Civilizations-Book
    Two
The History of Antediluvian Giants
The Antediluvian History of Earth
Ancient Underground Cities and
    Tunnels
Strange Objects Which Should Not Exist

Longevity Training-Book 4-Your Spiritual Connection

Strange and Ancient Places in the USA
A Theory of Ancient Prehistory And
      Giant Aliens
<u>Aliens and Space</u>
Aliens and Secret Technology
Aliens Are Already Among Us
Designing and Building Space Colonies
Humanity and the Universe

All About Moon Bases
All About Mars Journeys and Settlement
The Space and Aliens Six Books Bundle
A Theory of Ancient Prehistory and
      Giant Aliens
The Space Colonies and Space
      Structures Coloring Book
All About Asteroids

<u>The Longevity Training Series</u>

(A transcription of the online Multimedia Longevity Coaching Training Program)

The Personal Longevity Training Series-Book1-Long Lived Persons
The Personal Longevity Training Series-Book2-Your Soul's Purpose
The Personal Longevity Training Series-Book3-Enable Your Life Urge
The Personal Longevity Training Series-Book4-Your Spiritual Connection
The Personal Longevity Training Series-Book5-Having Love in Your Heart
The Personal Longevity Training Series-Book6-Energy Body Health
The Personal Longevity Training Series-Book7-The Science of Longevity
The Personal Longevity Training Series-Book8-Physical Body Health
The Personal Longevity Training Series-Book9-Avoiding Accidents
The Personal Longevity Training Series-Book10-Implementing These Principles

The Personal Longevity Training Series-Books One Thru Ten

These books are all available in digital and printed formats from my
website and on Amazon, Barnes & Noble, Apple ITunes, and many other sites

My Books Website is: http://mkettingtonbooks.com

Longevity Training-Book 4-Your Spiritual Connection

<u>Signup for our Mailing List to get the following:</u>

1) A discount coupon for 25% discount on all books on our site

2) Occasional Notices of new books available

3) Occasional Email on other offerings of ours (Monthly)

Go to this link to sign-up:

http://personal-longevity.com/mkebooks/emailsignup/

And click this link to get the FREE 102 page Ebook titled "Secrets of Many Things"

If you have any questions about this book or other subjects please contact the Author at:

mke@mkettingtonbooks.com

Longevity Training-Book 4-Your Spiritual Connection

Longevity Training-Book 4-Your Spiritual Connection

Longevity Training-Book 4-Your Spiritual Connection

Table of Contents

Longevity Training-Book 4-Your Spiritual Connection

Introduction

Back in 2008 I became very interested in the field of Longevity and Physical Immortality. After a lot of research this led me to my first book on the subject "Physical Immortality: A History and How to Guide". This book was pretty popular and I wanted to continue learning about Longevity and what things we could do about it in our lives.

The subject continued to fascinate me to the point that I developed a Longevity Coaching program over a couple of years starting in 2011. This online training program was multimedia—consisting of videos, my writings on longevity to read, online exercises, and tests for each of ten courses. It also included a lot of additional resources for each course including extra courses on how to become a successful Longevity Coach. A student who completed the training and tests successfully would become certified as a "Longevity Coach" and authorized to teach this material to others.

I developed a set of ten principles on longevity which are as follows:

The 10 Principles of Personal Longevity are:

- The Reality of Long Lived People
- Defining Your Purpose in Life
- Enabling the Life Urge
- Your Spiritual Health
- Having Love in Your Heart
- Energy Body Health
- The Science of Longevity
- Physical Body Health
- Using your Intuition for Safety
- Implementation of these principles

What are the 10 Principles all about?

The Reality of Long Lived People

The first principle is where I provide lots of evidence of people who have lived well over the age of 120 years old to 150-180-200, and even a 256 year old man from China:

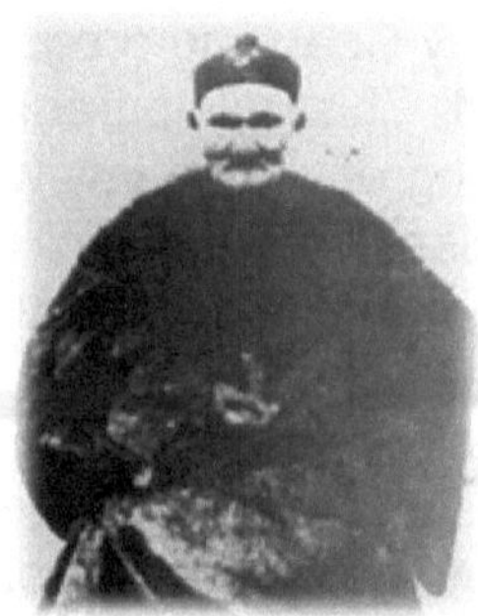

LI CHING-YUN: The Longest Lived person of record-256 Years (Source-The New York Times-May 6, 1933)

The Second Principle of Life Purpose

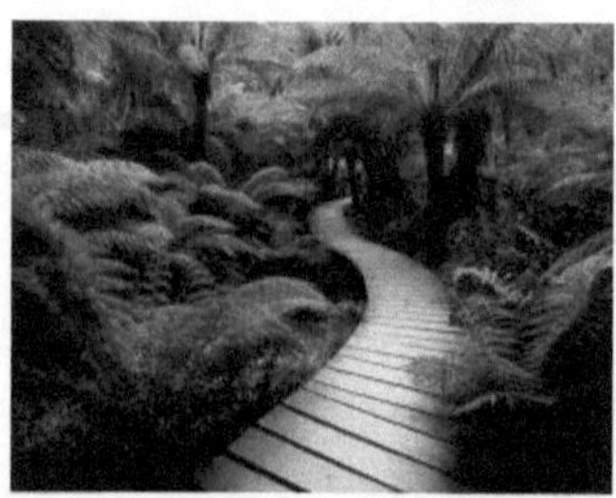

One of the things that occurred to me when I was putting the 10 principles together was that if one doesn't have a reason to live, or purpose in life--then what is the point?

This meant I had to add a very important step of how you can develop your own life purpose, or bring it up to date with your phase in life. Without reviewing your purpose-- then none of the rest of the principles matter.

Enabling the Life Urge

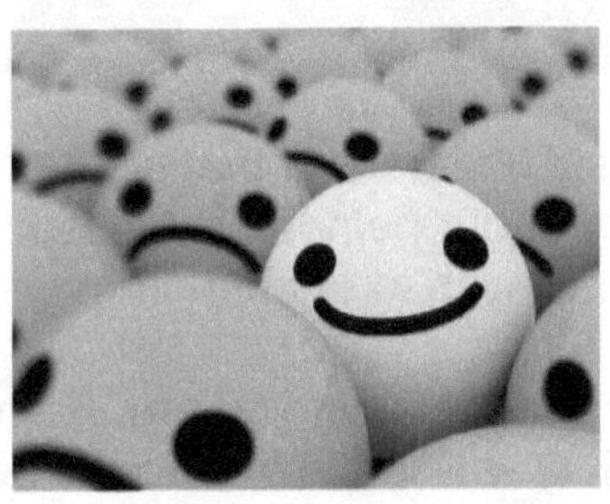

Have you ever realized how we are all programmed to expect to live through certain stages in life and then die? It's so common in our society that we don't think it odd that we expect to die at a certain age?

Have you ever heard radio ads saying "You are getting up in your sixties and seventies" so it's time to come out to our cemetery and buy a plot"

How ridiculous is this? And do you see how much our subconscious has been programmed towards death?

This principle is all about reprogramming ourselves to have a more positive outlook on life and its possibilities.

Having a Spiritual Connection in Your Life

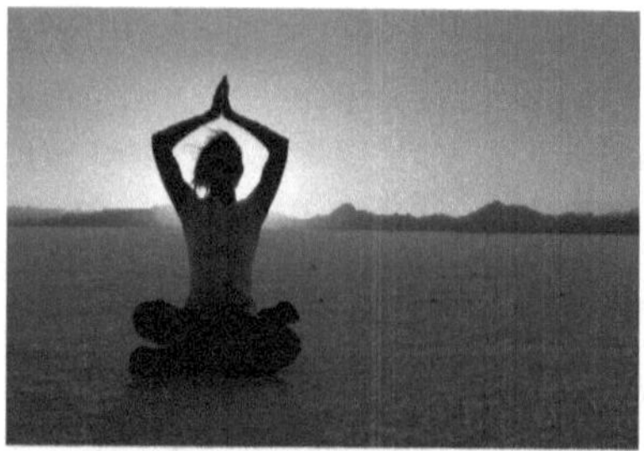

Most of us innately understand that we have a spiritual core in the center of our being. It is this spiritual core that we need to connect with to enable our physical health too.

It doesn't matter what religion you are. Regular meditation, deep prayer, or just walking in the woods helps you make and keep that connection in your life.

Having Love in Your Heart

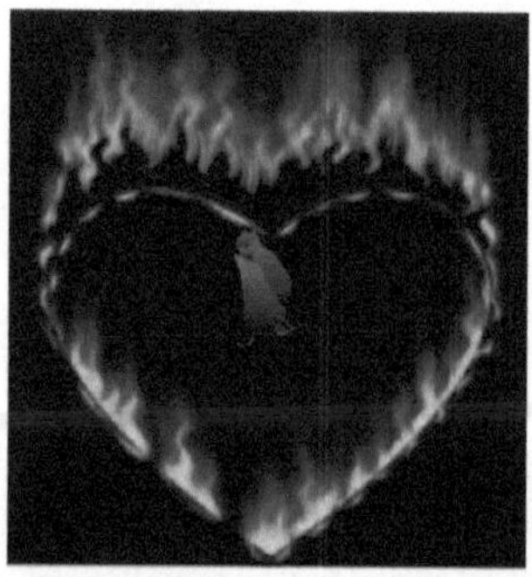

One of the most important things I learned in the last five years was that Unconditional Love is a real and physical thing. It is a powerful energy force in life and not just a philosophical belief system.

I considered it so important that I added it as a separate principle of longevity.

True Unconditional Love is healing, embodies happiness, and is a powerful part of our vital forces.

Energy Body Health

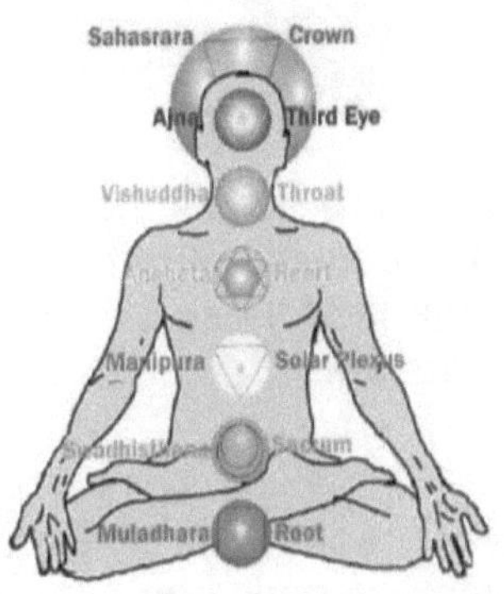

We all have an energy body which is part of our vital forces. The Indians talk about the "Chakras" and the Chinese talk about "Energy Meridians" in Acupuncture.

We should all learn different practices to keep our vital forces flowing for maximum health and vitality.

The Science of Longevity

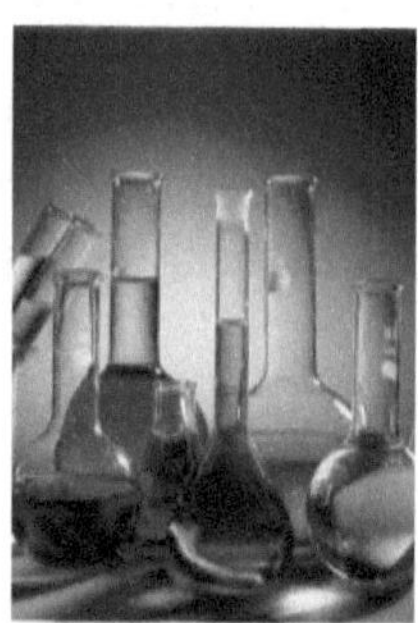

Science and Medicine are making new discoveries all the time that we can take advantage of to extend our lives. Why not take advantage of these discoveries which provide new therapies and supplements to increase our longevity.

There is also a lot we can learn from plants and animals. We all share the same genetic basis.

Some of these plants and animals live thousands of years and some cells are immortal.

What can we learn from them to apply to our lives?

Physical Body Health

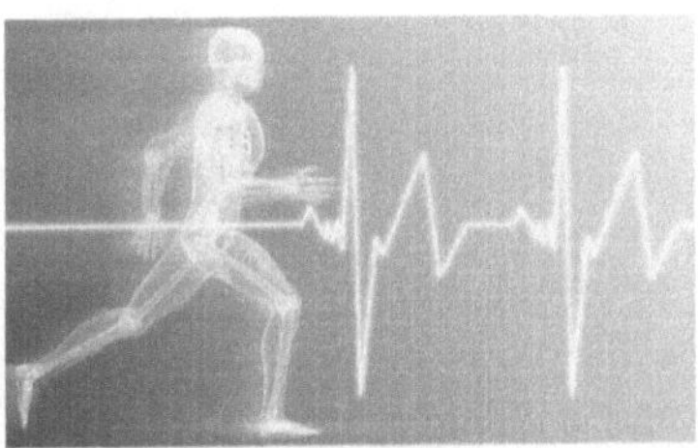

There are many types of supplements used for anti-aging for thousands of years. What can we learn about them that we can apply to our lives?

What other considerations about our physical health does nontraditional or alternative medicine offer?

Using Your Intuition for Safety

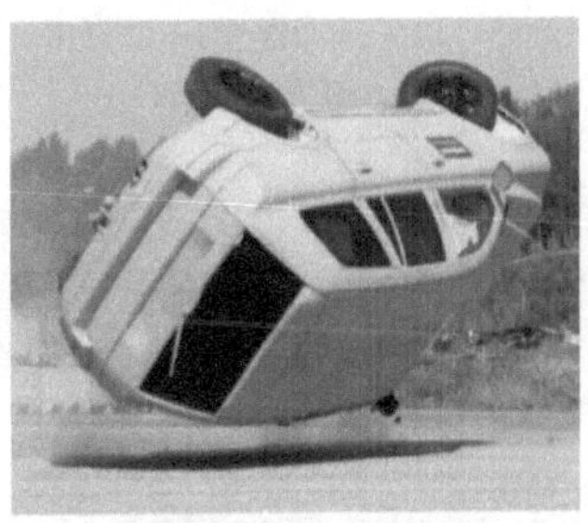

Once you have established your own long term health then what is the greatest danger you face?

ACCIDENTS

We can learn to use our intuition to make us safer as well as see potential future events which may be good too.

Why not open up to the possibilities of how our spirit has this natural ability in all of us?

Implementing These Principles in Your Life

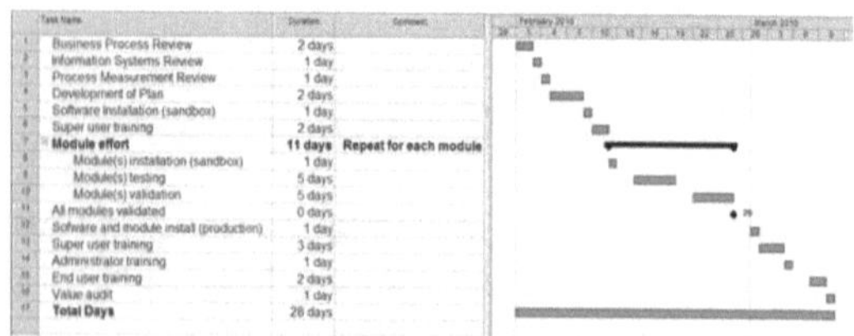

It's nice to read about all these concepts, but how can you really apply them to your own life?

This is what the chapter on implementation is all about, and it helps you plan a lifelong change in your health focus to live these principles and truly experience long term health, greater happiness, and extended longevity.

For five years I amended and improved these materials which now include a lot more information and helpful concepts for students wanting to improve their longevity and those of others.

I transcribed my videos and other materials to this book so you can read it all, and later hear it in an AudioBook.

This book is priced pretty inexpensively, compared to the online training and certification program which sells in total for $1,995 USD. If you are interested in taking the entire online program at a major discount, then please contact me at:

Marty@personal-longevity.com

Hope you enjoy these materials since when applied correctly they will significantly change your life.

PLP Concepts Overview

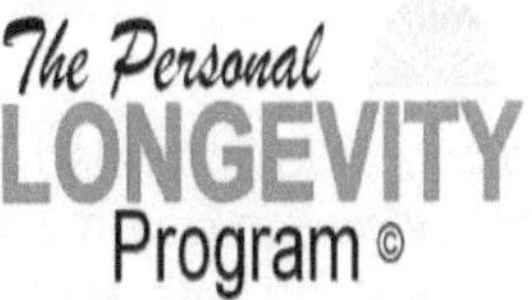

(Transcription of overview video)

Hello I'm Martin Ettington and I'd like to introduce you to the Personal Longevity Program which is an integrated holistic approach to long-term health. In this video we will only cover the high level concepts which comprise individual courses in the coaching certificate program for personal longevity.

The first concept is that long lived people exist and have existed for hundreds of thousands of years. We cover in the first course all about their records; along with people not only in places you might think like India, but in Europe and the United States-people who've lived long lives and well documented cases.

We discuss people who have lived well over the age of 120 and even the case of a Chinaman who lived to 256 years old. Plus a lot of mythology about people who have lived even longer lives so you get an idea that extending your life much longer than we think is currently medically and scientifically possible is certainly something that can happen.

The second course's concept has to do with finding your souls purpose. The point of wanting to live a long life is to know what your purpose in life is, so we go through some readings and some exercises to help you determine where soul's purpose in life is. Then doing goals as a fundamental concept so you will know the motivations in your life.

Third is the "Psychology of Living" also known by certain practitioners as "Removing the death Urge". The psychology of living has to do with seeking a positive image about your ability to live a long time. We tend to be programmed from birth about the idea that we are going to go through certain stages in our life as a child, as a teenager, and as adults. It's about reprogramming your subconscious as to the possibilities of a long life.

I've also learned in my life that it is very important to be able open your heart to unconditional love. When you're able to love unconditionally it also helps increase the strength of your immune system and fight off disease. So this is an aspect of spiritual growth. The courses also cover unconditional love and energy body forces. Managing your energy body is an important component of who you are in having energy working properly in your body and is another aspect of health for the length of longevity.

There are many types of scientific and medical research which are being done today and which will contribute to human longevity in the future.

Do you know that the average lifespan in the United States in 1900 was only about 40 years? We have doubled lifespan in the last century with current technologies but things under way in terms of scientific and medical improvements will help extend your lives further.

Also in this course on longevity we will cover a lot of the concepts which are being researched by scientists today. There are suggestions for more things you can do to do to use this science to improve your health along with physical supplements.

A unique thing that I thought about and decided to offer in these courses has to do with all my experiences in prophecy and how I was able to change outcomes on accidents that would occur to me by using simple exercises you can learn to change these outcomes. If you're in great health often the biggest thing you have to worry about are accidents.

We also provide guidelines you can follow on a daily basis and plans you can make to live healthier and happier and have a much longer life than you ever thought possible.

Thank you for listening !

Course #4 Intro Video

(Transcription of Video)

Hello this is Marty Ettington. I'd like to welcome you to course number four. In the spiritual program in this course, we're going to learn about how your spiritual health is the number one key to your longevity.

Your spiritual health is the number one thing you can do. The connection to your spirit being the number one thing you can do to improve your long-term health and be able to live a long life. Some of the concepts you will learn here include how your spiritual, your energy, and your physical bodies all synchronize together to give you a long-term health. And that working on each of those is critical to achieving that. The power in terms of spirituality we're talking about is the enlightenment process and the importance of stillness.

The ability to be still and connect to your spirit which lives in the timeless space-less realm is key to having that connection spirituality to bring stillness down into your being. To bring that light force of the spirit down into your being which helps keep the reality of stillness can be shown by different examples from science. For instance, most physicists think of the Big Bang and how it created universe. That's a very popular thing that's known about the universe-that everything was created all at once from a single point. Time and space came from Big Bang. Before that here was no time or space what there was-was a timeless space-less realm-which many of the Eastern Yogi's would say is the same as the realm of the Spirit.

Additionally have you ever heard of the term "Black Hole"? A Black hole refers to a star which is larger than a certain size and when it runs out of energy it collapses to a point. So inside the black hole there is no time or space-again a timeless space-less realm. In addition science like quantum mechanics has had a lot of experiments in recent years that prove that there's action at a distance without intervening space; more evidence of a timeless space-less realm. From all my experience, This I believe is the realm of the spirit. The consciousness that is behind a universe that we all have a piece of within us, So the goal of this course is to help you find stillness. Help people learn what it's all about and the importance of it. And you can find stillness in different religions. For instance like the Protestant church behind me or it can be through specific actions that you take by yourself like meditation. If you've never meditated that's something you should learn to do.

We'll do an exercise involved with that learning different types of prayer to help you center yourself or even things like just walking in the woods and feeling one with nature can be a spiritual experience too. So again to get one thing out of this course is that the key to long-term health and longevity is having good spiritual health and becoming center in the spirit. And that's what we're going to go into in this course. I hope you enjoy it and don't forget to take the test at the end the course because that will be a part of your certification process for the personal longevity program. Thank you. Talk to you soon.

Your Whole Being

(Extracts of Chapters 8a-d and Chapter 10 from "Physical Immortality: A History and How to Guide")

Chapter 8: Your Spiritual, Energy, & Physical Bodies

One of the key concepts in this book is that you are not just your physical body.

These are concepts which are woven into many religions and philosophies, with related energy body concepts mostly being understood in the East more than the West.

Many believe that your entire being consists of at least three states as described below.

a.   The Spirit

Here we mean the spirit which is your "soul" or core of your being. An individual's spirit is one with the God spirit and is present in every person and every being. It exists outside of time and space. This is a place some call "no time and no space". It is everywhere present simultaneously.

The spirit exists in all things and each person has that same core spirit within them.

We can learn to live focused more in the spirit through a variety of religious, meditational, and philosophical traditions.

b.   The Energy Body

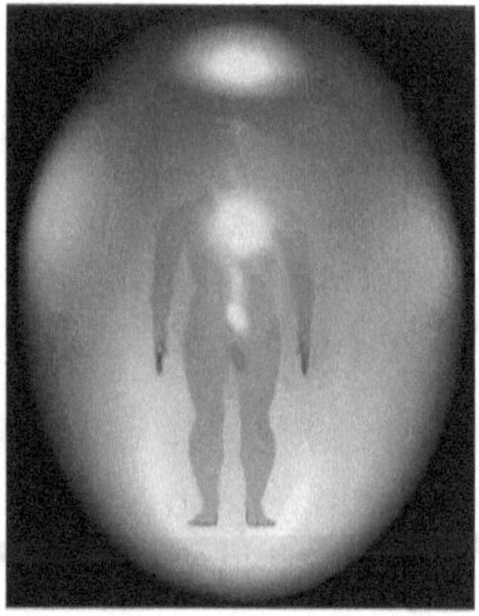

Figure 4-An artist's rendering of a Full Body

Some organizations like the Hindus and Theosophists believe we have multiple energy body levels. The Theosophists (9) believe there are at least six distinct energy bodies. Many other traditions only talk about one energy body which provides the life force to energize our physical bodies.

The acupuncture meridians and chakras are all parts of the energy body which exists in very close proximity to the physical body.

The aura is also a manifestation of the energy body too, which overlaps your physical body.

Many people claim to be able to see "auras" including this Author. The aura is the physical energy manifestation of the energy body. All living people have an aura and one can tell a lot about their health by how their aura looks.

c.   The Physical Body

This is the body most of us know, and that most of us think is all of us that exists. This is the body we want to heal and energize to achieve physical immortality.

Exercises done on the physical body also affect the energy body.

Herbal supplements work from the physical body to help correct energy flows in your energy body.

d.   How the Bodies Work Together

The concept of the spiritual development exercises, and physical exercises in this book is that they help increase the synchronization of these bodies.

By bringing the absolute peace and stillness of the spirit down into the energy and physical bodies you increase the perfection and health of those bodies.

This is since in the normal course of events the stresses of our life cause more randomness or entropy in our energy and physical bodies. These stresses of daily life age us prematurely and cause disease.

We can repair our energy and physical bodies by integrating them better with the spiritual body; and getting the energies to flow in the correct patterns, chakras, and meridians, and with more vital force.

Chapter 10: Spiritual Growth Practices

This chapter is intended as a guide to some of the spiritual practices which can be used to make your physical body healthier and younger.

It is not an exclusive list since I'm sure there are many paths which all go to enlightenment; with immortality as a side benefit.

In fact, the goal of spiritual growth should be enlightenment—not immortality. However, since immortality is the subject of this book I'm really focusing on a side effect of the spiritual development process.

a.   The Importance of Stillness

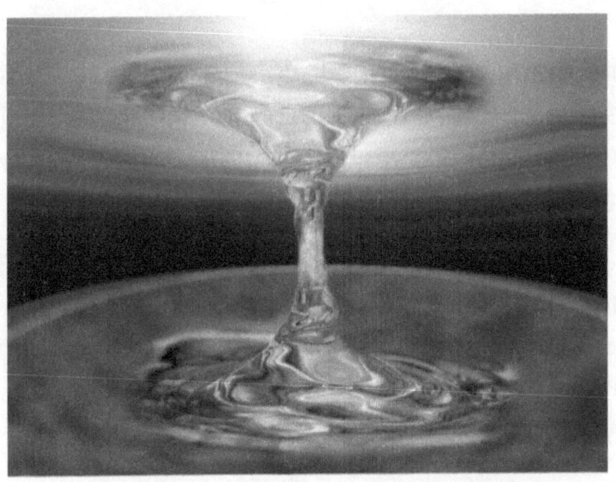

Figure 5-Water frozen in time-Stillness

How does spiritual growth help one stay healthy; and what is stillness?

The ideas I'm going to discuss here relate to eastern Asian concepts of the spirit as taught mainly in China and India.

Buddhism, Taoism, Zen, and other eastern religions and philosophies all teach that the spirit is the core of our being; and that our physical bodies are just an extension of that spirit into the physical level of existence.

By learning to let your mind or ego release its hold on the illusion of our current existence, we become aware of the spirit behind or at the core of our being. This spirit is the pure oneness of God and exists in no time and no space. (A concept which we really can't envision with our minds or egos only).

There are many techniques taught to get closer to realizing the core of a person's being. These techniques all involve practicing spiritual growth, love, and/or meditation with a goal of enlightenment.

There are thousands of books and practices on this subject so I will not try to duplicate them in this short synopsis.

The Chinese stress that the stillness and oneness obtained through spiritual growth are one of the main keys to keeping the body healthy for a long life. Many Taoist techniques and teachings stress the achievement of "stillness" as a prelude to physical immortality.

The stillness I'm referring to is found mainly through meditation. In Christian terms it is often referred to as the "Peace that passes all understanding".

It is hard to describe the feeling of stillness since it is like when you first wake up in the morning after a deep sleep—but even quieter and deeper.

The feeling of stillness has a strong effect on your body—it seems to make the randomness of your cells quiet down into a more restful state.

Meditation is taught many places, I've even found a company called Holosync which sells CDs that help even beginners achieve deep states of relaxation that usually takes advanced Yogis years of practice.

Stillness is not something achieved overnight but takes years, (even with modern advanced CD techniques) to start showing results.

However, the effects of stillness practices probably have the most profound effects on your body's aging as anything else recommended in this book.

This is since as you start to achieve stillness, your Ego is realizing its core is really part of the spirit—not a separate mind. The spirit exists outside time and space. This connection with your spirit has a profound health effect on the body in terms of peace and well-being.

When meditating in this state you can feel stillness penetrating your body.

It feels like your body is reaching a relaxed state never realized; even in sleep.

The state of the stillness of your spirit provides a modified blueprint for your body's health.

It is a lot of work to set aside time every day to meditate. The good news is you will find that after some weeks of practicing, this time becomes something you look forward to. This is since meditation is so relaxing it becomes a way to recharge you for daily activities in the world.

I also find that meditation makes my mind more alert when I wake up in the morning and gives me a sharper intellectual edge at work.

b.   The Reality of Stillness

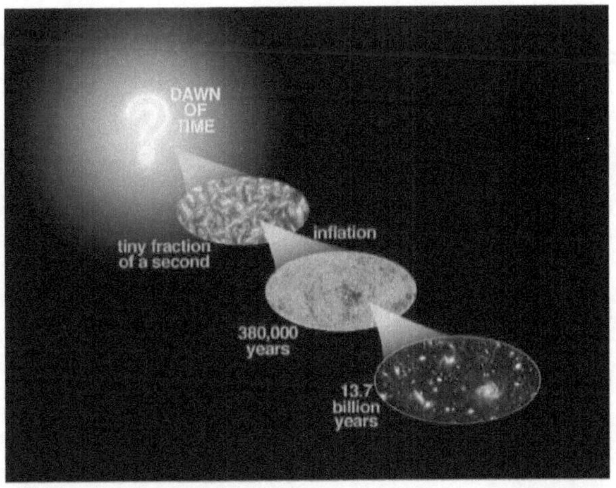

Figure 6-The growth of the Universe

Most people believe that God was the initial creative force which started the Universe.

Physicists and Astronomers all agree that the Universe we know was created from nothing and inflated in a huge explosion called the "Big Bang". As it inflated time and space as we know them came into existence.

When you study Einstein's Relativistic physics you being to understand that time and space are inextricably linked.
You can't have one without the other.

Given our understanding of physics, we know that time and space didn't exist before the Big Bang. The state of things before creation then was "No Time & No Space".

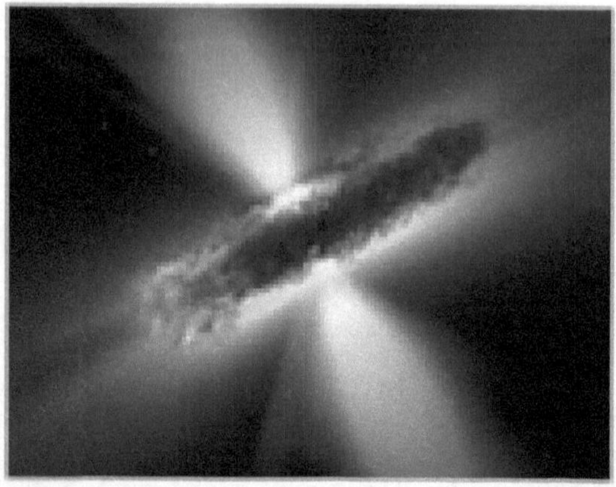

Figure 7-A notional picture of a black hole

Another subject of great interest to astrophysicists is what are called "Black Holes". Black Holes are a result of Einstein's equations and astronomers have verified their existence in the last few decades.

Black Holes are stars which due to their own mass have collapsed down to an infinitely small point and where time stops. Scientists do not understand where all that mass goes.

Hmm…. A   Black Hole seems to be another example of part of reality that exists without time and space.

In Quantum Physics, time is also viewed differently than we perceive it on a daily basis. Here is a quote from a Physics website explaining this view:

The upshot is that, on the microscopic level, there is no direction to time -- and this is even more spectacularly true in quantum physics than in classical physics. In the microscopic domain, everything just exists in a kind of nebulous, atemporal continuum. Then, every once in a while, something becomes observable, and enters the one-dimensional time continuum. The arrow of time does not exist in the universe as a whole. It only exists in individual subjective views of the universe!

I think it is fair to say that the place of stillness where time and space don't exist is part of our reality.

Therefore, it shouldn't be considered too strange that our immortal spirit is part of and one with that stillness.

c.   Finding Stillness in Major Religions

Christianity is the largest religion in the world, and one I know pretty well since I was raised in Methodist and Presbyterian churches growing up. I also attended multiple churches as an adult and participated in Bible study groups for a number of years.

Prayer is the key to stillness as a Christian. There are many books on Prayer and Prayer techniques. One needs to focus on spirit and becoming one with the spirit to move towards a state of stillness as a Christian.

The fact that so many of the long lived persons recorded in this book lived in Christian cultures probably indicates that being a devoted Christian can help you "live in the spirit" as much as many other spiritual techniques.

I'm not as familiar with Judaism and Islam, but the same approach applies in doing prayers in those religions.

The key to Prayer in your religion or spiritual approach is that you must learn to focus on the spirit of God which is inside you; and is the core of your being. That spirit exists in eternal peace; outside of time and space.

Once you learn to focus on that spirit in your prayer you will be able to bring that peace and stillness into your physical body to calm it and provide more health.

d.   Biblical Quotes Relating to Stillness and the Spirit

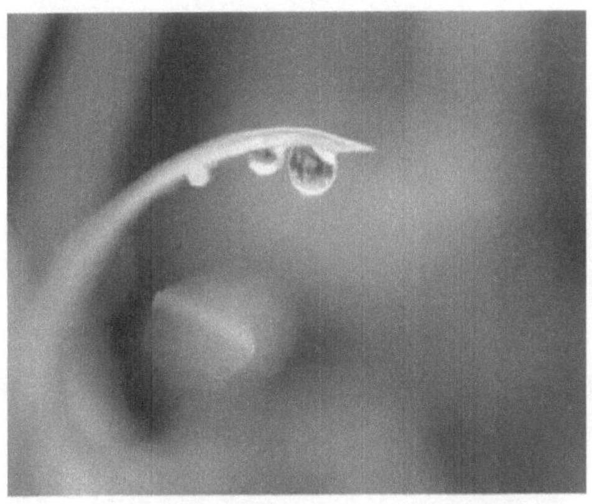

Figure 8-Morning Stillness

Here are a number of Biblical quotes which relate to the power of the spirit and the state of stillness (peace) I've described above.

•   You will experience God's peace which is far more wonderful than the   human mind can understand. His peace will keep your thoughts and your   hearts quiet and at rest as you trust in Jesus Christ. (Philippians 4:7 LB)

•   He will keep in perfect peace all those who trust in him, whose thoughts turn often to the Lord. (Isaiah 26:3 LB)

•   The work of righteousness shall be peace; and the effect of righteousness,   quietness and assurance forever. (Isaiah 32:17 KJV)

- "You shall receive power when the Holy Spirit has come upon you; and you   shall be my witnesses both in Jerusalem, and in all Judea and Samaria,   and even to the remotest part of the Earth. (Acts 1:8 NASB)

- For by one Spirit are we all baptized into one body (1 Corinthians 12:13 KJV)

- I will ask the Father and he will give you another Comforter, and he will   never leave you. He is the Holy Spirit. The spirit who leads into all truth.   The world at large cannot receive him; for it isn't looking for him and   doesn't recognize him. But you do, for he lives with you now, and some day   shall be in you. (John 14:16,17 LB)

- Do you not know that you are a temple of God and that the spirit of God   dwells within you? (1 Corinthians 3:16 NASB)

There are many more quotes about the spirit of God, but the key is that they all relate to that core of God's spirit inside us all.

e.   Golden Rules to Live Forever

Harry Gaze was a Philosopher and Teacher back in the early 20th Century. He was a teacher and lecturer in practical Metaphysics, New Thought, and Divine Science. He began his lecture work as early as 1898 and published numerous books on Metaphysics.

His book titled "How to Live Forever with Golden Rules for Successful Living" is very relevant to our study of physical immortality, and was first published in 1905. (He also wrote an earlier work on the subject in 1904 titled "How to Live Forever, The Science and Practice").

Like some other writers on the subject of unlimited longevity he believed that growing old and the body decaying was not inevitable! His belief was that the power of the spirit and thought on the body could keep one young forever.

Harry believed in several principles which guided his thinking:

a) The body literally and completely returns to dust in less than one year, and during this period, a new body is constructed molecule by molecule.
b)   Conscious cooperation with this change is the secret to eternal youth.
c)   Old age and somatic death are brought about by conditions which can be   effectually prevented.

He had a set of Golden Rules for Eternal Youth which are reproduced here:

1.	*Golden Rule for Eternal Youth Number One*: Realize there is one divine life in which you live, move, and have your being.

2.	*Golden Rule for Eternal Youth Number Two*: Realize that as a Son of God you are heir to God's immortality here and now; claim your birthright.

3.	*Golden Rule for Eternal Youth Number Three*: Realize that your body is a template of the Holy Spirit.

4.	*Golden Rule for Eternal Youth Number Four:* Deeply realize that your body is an expression of your mind, and attune yourself to infinite spirit.

5.	*Golden Rule for Eternal Youth Number Five:* Realize that by virtue of molecular renewal, which is constantly in operation, your body is constantly made new.

6.	*Golden Rule for Eternal Youth Number Six:* Keep in mind that nature's constant renewal of the body gives the opportunity of building a better body with each succeeding renewal.

7.	*Golden Rule for Eternal Youth Number Seven:* Practice rhythmical breathing and freely use your diaphragm, the organ that is the muscular floor of your upper internal organs, and the ceiling of your lower organs.

8.   *Golden Rule for Eternal Youth Number Eight:*
Realize that eternal youth is   harmony and positive
cooperation with the upward law of continuous   growth
and the law of attraction.

9.   *Golden Rule for Eternal Youth Number Nine:*
Realize that the secret of   eternal youth is cooperation
with God in creative, individual, volitional   evolution.

10.   *Golden Rule for Eternal Youth Number Ten:*
Practice faithfully the daily   affirmations for Eternal
Youth, doing them in a regular, cumulative   sequence.

11.   *Golden Rule for Eternal Youth Number Eleven:*
Practice concentrative   exercises daily, and develop
control of attention and thought selectivity.   Also do
meditative exercises and the Silence.

12.   *Golden Rule for Eternal Youth Number Twelve:*
Realize the oneness of   your inner Christ life with
God, thinking of God as an Infinite Life, Infinite   Power,
Infinite Health, Infinite Youth, Infinite Peace, Infinite Joy.

Note the focus on meditation in Rule Eleven. This was a
very unusual term to use one hundred years ago and
indicates some familiarity with knowledge from the East.

Rule number 10 mentions the daily affirmations for Eternal
Youth. These are listed below too. Mr. Gaze recommends
practicing one daily for the whole month, then starting over
again:

1)   Adaptation: Whenever essential, I adapt myself readily to more perfect   change.
2)   Adjustment: I give myself freely to wise, spiritual, mental, and physical adjustment.
3)   Beauty: I realize that the beauty of enduring youth is as deep as the   innermost recesses of the soul.
4)   Buoyancy: In every thought, nerve, and muscle I express the perfect   buoyancy of joyous youth.
5)   Confidence: I cheerfully react to all conditions with the boundless
          confidence of youth.
6)   Courage: I increasingly attain the natural courage of strong and vital youth.
7)   Creativeness: The Divine Spirit, everywhere, and in and through me,   inspires me with keen creativeness.
8)   Daring: I blend the pure daring of youth with the wisdom of growth and   experience.
9)   Elasticity: My sense of freedom and flexibility of mind find its   correspondence in bodily elasticity.
10)   Energy: My whole being is vitally energized with the radiant life of the   Divine Spirit.
11)   Flexibility: I joyously affirm the quality of flexibility in every cell, muscle and   artery of my being.
12)   Freshness: Bathing in the commonness of pure spirit, I am fresh as the   dawn of day.
13)   Gracefulness: By wise exercise, relaxation, visualization and nourishment,   I maintain the gracefulness of youth.
14)   Happiness: I realize that the true spring of happiness is within me.
15)   Initiative: The spirit of initiative and wise adventure freely motivates and   activates me.
16)   Joy: The joy of eternal youth is my daily light and inspiration.

17)   Loveliness: The loveliness of ever-renewing youth is the expression of   loving and lovable qualities.
18)   Newness: Every day and every moment, my body is being made new in every cell, molecule and atom.
19)   Optimism: I look joyously forward with the spirit of youthful optimism.
20)   Progressiveness: I am a progressive conscious, purposeful and individual factor in my evolution.
21)   Purity: I see life with the eyes of child like purity blended with power and poise.
22)   Radiance: I am radiant with the light, life and love of infinite wisdom.
23)   Receptivity: Knowing that I am a child of God, I am at all times receptive to the highest inspiration.
24)   Rejuvenation: I am devoted and consecrated to all habits that rejuvenate and heal.
25)   Renewal: I am an ever-renewing and ever-unfolding expression of infinite life.
26)   Responsiveness: As the years unfold, I maintain my full, free responsiveness to the best in life.
27)   Unfoldment: I am open, receptive and responsive to new growth and unfoldments.
28)   Versatility: I joyously express the creative spirit in me in the versatility that unites youth with experience.
29)   Vitality: I think, speak, breathe, exercise, relax and nourish my mind and body for increasing vitality.
30)   Youth: I realize that the fountain of Eternal Youth, like the Kingdom of God, is here and now, within me.
31)   Zest: My thought, speech and action are all radiantly animated with youthful zest for living.

f.   The Importance of Love

Having a lot of LOVE in your life is also important to living a long one.

Many studies have shown that being married will give you a longer average lifetime by several years than persons who remain single their whole lives.

Love is of many types-physical and spiritual; and has multiple aspects.

Our spirit is one with the universe; and is the animating force of all life. Therefore, it makes a lot of sense that the more love we have in our lives, the more we are living in the spirit and synchronizing our spirit with our energy and physical bodies.

Although you may often think your family is stressful and can sometimes be annoying, just remember that these relationships are providing a positive impact on you for the long term.

Just remember the loving kindness most families and close circles of friends exhibit to each other is something which is a core part of a healthy life on earth.

Becoming a hermit is not required to be physically immortal and probably a hindrance.

g.   A Positive Outlook on Life

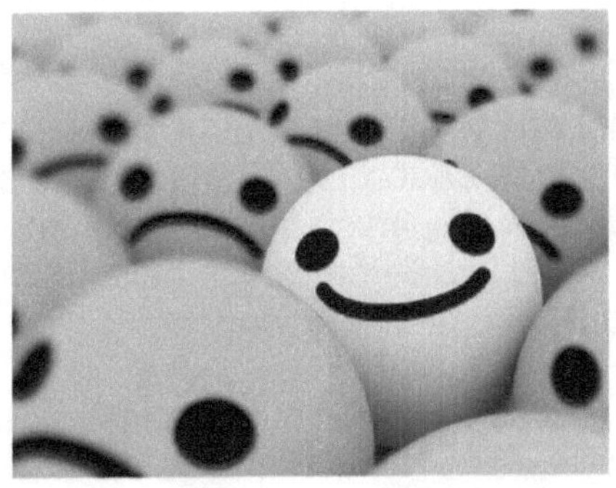

Figure 9-Do you stand out in the crowd?

How does a positive outlook on life increase your life span?

Optimism and a positive outlook increases our vitality and spiritual connections.

If you are positive you have a better chance of extracting yourself from an unhealthful or dangerous situation.

An article extract from an M.D. reinforces the importance of a positive outlook:

> "Optimism is necessary for good health," says Charles L. Raison, MD, a psychiatrist and director of the behavioral immunology clinic at Emory University School of Medicine in Atlanta. "There's growing evidence that, for many medical illnesses, stress and a negative mental state -- pessimism, feeling overwhelmed, being burnt out -- has a

negative effect on immunity, which is especially important in rheumatoid arthritis."

Indeed, your brain can create all sorts of tailor-made prescriptions to nurture your body. Raison says these include endorphins -- the natural painkillers; gamma globulin, which fortifies your immune system; and interferon, which helps combat infections, viruses, even cancer.

When depression sets in, we're less likely to take care of ourselves, which means the brain doesn't get prompted to produce those great natural remedies, Raison says. We don't exercise, because we don't have much energy. We don't eat right. We lose sleep -- or we sleep too much.

i.   The Yoga Sutras of Patanjali

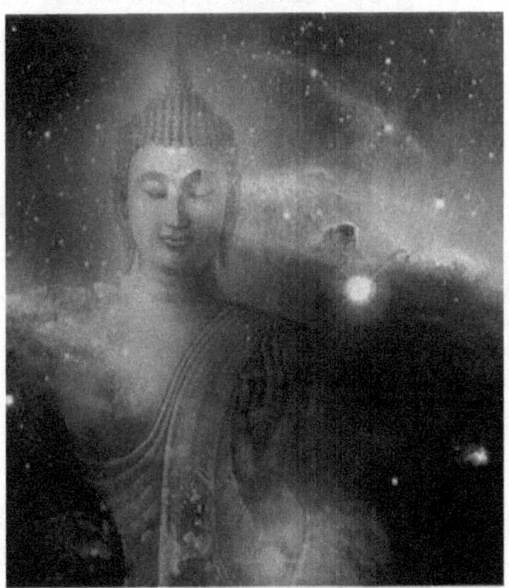

Figure 10-A Notional Picture of a Yogic Adept

This book was written in Sanskrit and is one of the great spiritual works of India. It is available in print on the Internet. It describes the path to enlightenment and attainment of spiritual powers. The Sutras were written over 2,000 years ago by some estimates.

The Sutras are often described as a scientific exposition on the science of yoga and consists of 4 books with numerous translations in English.

Although the Sutras don't talk specifically of physical immortality, the powers available as a result of the spiritual development process would also affect the body in a very positive manner.

In Book 3, Sutra 45 we have an example of what I'm referring to regarding spiritual powers from the process of enlightenment. This would probably cause a lot of longevity in the physical body if exercised properly:

Book 3 Sutra 45-Thereupon will come the manifestation of the atomic and other powers, which are the endowment of the body, together with its unassailable force.

An exposition of this sutra is as follows:

> *The body in question is, of course, the etheric body of the spiritual man. He is said to possess eight powers: the atomic, the power of assimilating himself with the nature of the atom, which will, perhaps, involve the power to disintegrate material forms; the power of levitation; the power of limitless extension; the power of boundless reach, so that, as the commentator says, "he can touch the moon with the tip of his finger"; the power to accomplish his will; the power of gravitation, the correlative of levitation; the power of command; the power of creative will. These are the endowments of the spiritual man. Further, the spiritual body is unassailable. Fire burns it not, water wets it not, the sword cleaves it not, dry winds parch it not. And, it is said, the spiritual man can impart something of this quality and temper to his bodily vesture.*

Many forms of Yoga exist to develop one along the path. These include Raja, Gnana, Prana, Tantric, and other forms of Yoga.

Yoga teachers for many of these disciplines can be found in many major and minor cities around the world.

j.   A Course in Miracles

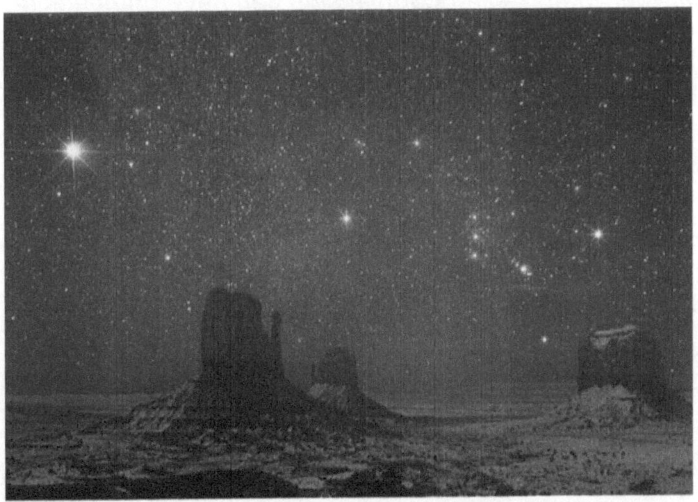

Figure 11-Infinite Spirit and Stillness

I would be remiss to end this section on Spiritual Growth without mentioning "A Course in Miracles" which has been published and disseminated since 1975 by the Foundation for Inner Peace.

The best explanation of the course comes from their website:

This is a course in miracles. It is a required course. Only the time you take it is voluntary. Free will does not mean that you can establish the curriculum.   It means only that you can elect what you want to take at a given time. The course does not aim at teaching the meaning of love, for that is beyond what can be taught. It does aim, however, at removing the blocks to the awareness of love's presence, which is your natural inheritance. The opposite of love is fear, but what is all-encompassing can have no opposite.

This course can therefore be summed up very simply in this way:

Nothing real can be threatened. Nothing unreal exists.

Herein lies the peace of God.

I did the course for about six months and found it was an excellent tool to help me become more centered and develop more stillness.

I had often felt in recent years that old thoughts, fears, and stresses were building up in my mind like dirt or crud, and were causing my spirit to be covered by a fog or cotton candy which made me less clear and not able to think as well.

One day I remember I was working on the Course in Miracles lessons and suddenly it felt like a large part of this shell of mentally accreted garbage suddenly came apart and sloughed off my spirit. It was a physical experience. An analogy might be a heavy coat of dirt and grime coming off a car after a good wash so that the bright colors and shininess of the car comes through again.

This course is another tool for spiritual growth which can help you get better connected to your spiritual core as part of the physical immortality process.

k.   Visualizing your Immortal Future

The key to visualizing your physically immortal future is not to imagine that you will get there but to imagine that you are already there. The more vividly you can imagine being immortal now and what you are doing very vividly, the more this changes the probability of your future to make it so.

Here is an excellent exercise to help your visualize yourself in health and happiness in your own immortal future:

a)   Relax for 5-10 minutes.
b)   Choose a happy scene of family, friends, or profession or activities that you want to visualize.
c)   We are going to picture the scene you have chosen at different ages. These ages will be 100, 200, and 500 years old. As you visualize you will be in that scene. You make it real. You will put energy and will into it to make it happen.
d)   You are now 100 years old. You are in the scene. People and scenery   are around you. You can feel the temperature; the light in the sky or   ceiling. You also smell the scene and you see everything vividly. You can
        look around and see details such as trees or on buildings or walls, etc.
e)   Your body feels healthy and you can tell you are youthful. Your solid   belief in your own immortality has been paying off for a while now.
f)   You are now 200 years old and it's the 23rd century. (Your lifestyle may have changed to something which is an earlier period in a place where change is slower).

Again, see your surroundings very vividly in a scene you enjoy. Feel all five senses. What do you see? What do you hear? What do you smell? What do you taste? What do you feel?

g)   You are now 500 years old and it's the 25th century. You may have travelled out   into the solar system or to a planet around another star. Life goes on and you are in a community of other immortals who have similar interests to you. Maybe you are getting educated for a new profession, or maybe you are an artist in a mode you never tried before. You have probably learned to teleport yourself by this time and live totally in the now. Look around you to see what's there. You feel very strong and   healthy as you usually do, and you have now been healthy and physically stable for centuries.

h)   Keep doing this imagery consistently every day for a few minutes until you start to feel solidity and that the events will happen. This is when you know that your will and energy have created the future.

You might want to record this visualization on tape to play back to yourself. Your own voice is the most powerful voice you can hear.

Mindfulness

Meditation and the Autonomic Nervous System

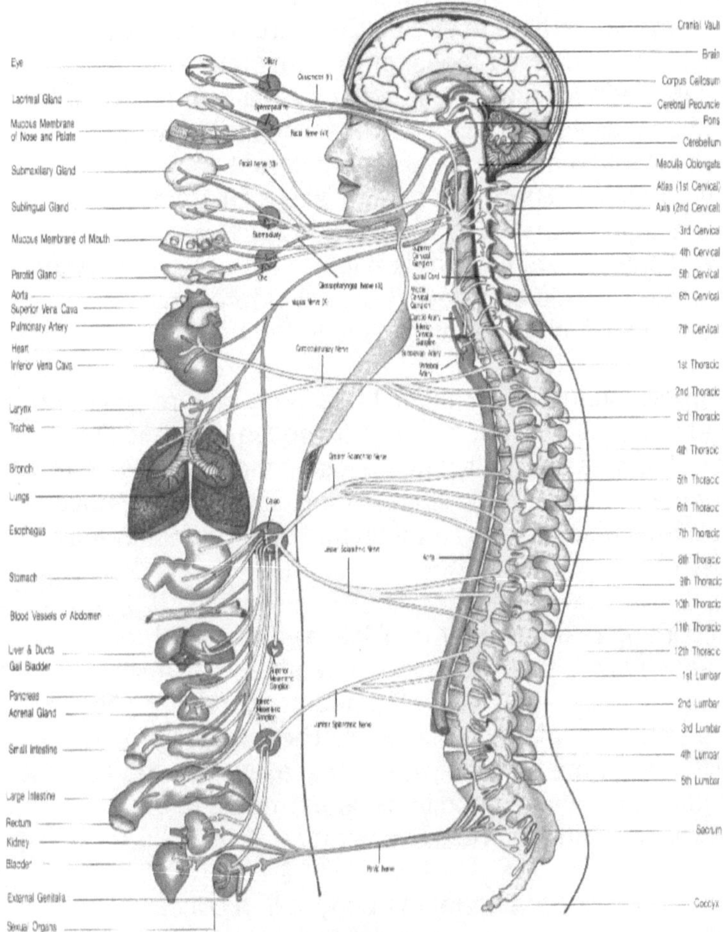

Aging is a health continuum. It is a delicate balance between nutrition and healing versus body deterioration.

As the body ages, the function of the cells in the body decline at various rates. As cell function declines, cells become vulnerable to stress. Cell "stress" includes processed and fatty foods, environmental toxins, poor sleep, negative life stress (both physical and emotional) , and excessive weight gain. Stressors illicit slow and chronic inflammation. There are different types of inflammation. There is a healthy acute inflammatory reaction in response to injury which starts and maintains the repair process. There is another type of inflammation which is chronic and slow. This is a different type of response which causes damage to the body.

Chronic inflammation plays a role in premature cell death and the development of chronic disease. Chronic Disease is defined as a long-lasting condition that can be controlled but not cured. Chronic illnesses include diabetes, obesity, heart disease, cancer, arthritis and other autoimmune diseases.

According to the Center for Disease Control, chronic disease is the leading cause of death and disability in the United States and 75% of US health care dollar goes to the treatment of these diseases. The number of individuals with one or more chronic diseases, as well as the cost for treatment of these conditions, is estimated to dramatically increase during the next five years.

Some sources state that the body is in a constant inflammatory state and that the individual can decrease the rate of cell aging thru lifestyle. Nutrition and physical activity are both very important. Our genes also play a role.

The organs in the body are controlled by the autonomic nervous system (ANS).

The ANS controls involuntary actions (such as heart beat, digestion) and is made of the nerves that relax the body [Parasympathetic Nervous System (PNS)] and nerves that respond to stress [Sympathetic Nervous System (SNS)]. There is a balance between the PNS and SNS. For the body to be in a good autonomic nervous state, the PNS should be more active than the SNS. The control station of the ANS is the brain.

The stressors that promote inflammation, also negatively affect the ANS. This imbalance can be improved by nutrition, physical activity and spiritual practices, such as meditation and prayer.

An example of the potential powerful effect of meditation has been demonstrated by a male client of the group. He is in his late 50's, has Diabetes Type 2, arthritis of a hip and is obese. He meditates daily and has been working with meditation for many years. Despite the negative stressors his body is confronted with, his ANS was in perfect balance. As the ANS affects every organ in the body this is a great basis for any life style improvement.

Meditation Introduction

(Transcription of Video)

Hello this is Marty Ettington and I want to welcome you to this introductory meditation video. This meditation video can be used as a resource for yourself or your clients to teach them the basics of meditation. There are many meditations you can get off the internet like YouTube but I thought I should include at least one basic meditation video in the training program-so here we go.

First I'd like you to sit down or lie down and close your eyes and start to relax. We're going to go through a relaxation procedure for our entire bodies to help take us down into a deeper relaxed state. First of all I'd like you to feel your left foot tighten-your foot tighten, your toes relax. We're going to do this for every part of your body. Now go to your left leg. Go up to feel the calf. See all the pressures on it; tensions-and up to your left knee and above the knee. Your thigh-feel all of that area and how it feels in your body.

Now tighten it up tight-tight-tight-relax now. Let's go to your right leg, your right foot. Tighten those toes and I mean really tight. Feel your foot-feel the tensions on your foot. Now let it go and start to learn the difference between relaxed parts of your body. Feel your body pulling up your right leg-your calf up to your knee. How the knee feels the joints and the thigh. The rest of your leg tightens up. Your legs tighten up that right leg. Let it go-let it go as you become more relaxed. Now start feeling the tensions on your bottom. The lower part of your body-how that feels.

The pressure the clothes-everything. Fill that sensation with peace. Tighten up your bottom-going further up to your chest and your lungs. Feel the heartbeat. Feel the air pumping out of your chest. Now take a breath tight-tight-tighten your chest. Everything's tightened-let it go now. Let's do the left arm. Take your hand-then your fists-You can feel your wrist relax now. The entire arm up to your elbow-the upper arm-let go.

Now we go to the right side. Close your right hand-make that fist tight-let go now. The rest of the arm-tighten it up. Tighten it up. Relax. Then come up to your neck-move your head around. Tighten your neck muscles. Now make them your neck tight-let it go. And we come up to the head. Facial muscles. Feel your facial muscles or cheeks-your ears.

On your whole face-relax now. Your body should be getting very relaxed. You want to let it go and become more relaxed. Now we're going to relax the mind. Your eyes are still closed. We're going to start a countdown process from10 to 1. I want you to feel that you're in warm water in a well or the ocean. It's very calm and peaceful and now we're going to start sinking. 10 we're starting to sink below the surface but we can still breathe everything The light is getting a little darker. 9 we're going deeper-yet deeper into the water. It's calm and peaceful. 8 sinking down more-sinking into the water-calmer and more peaceful. 7 sinking down-is getting darker and darker it's very relaxed. You're in a very relaxed happy place. 6 yet deeper. 5 it's very dark now-sinking-very peaceful. 3 calm and centered calm and centered too-very deep and peaceful. 1 now we're in a very dark-very deep-relaxed place. I just want to feel what's going on. Just feel it in your mind-is relaxed-let everything go. This is starting to become a meditative or deep prayer state.

Now let's visualize some things we want to happen-our connections from above and below. So I want you to start visualizing your connection from the base your spine down into the earth. Red light grounding you to the Earth. You feel very stable and energy is coming up from the Earth into your spine. And energizing you-but still you're very relaxed and very deep. Red energy comes up through your body and as it does you feel healthier and stronger-and more grounded both physically, and mentally. It comes up through your body all the way up to your head. Feel now-there's a white light that is coming down from above. The light of the spirit of God. It's coming into the top of your head-what we call the crown chakra-you can feel that brilliant white energy bringing health and love and spirituality as it courses down through your body from your head down from your neck. Into your body- it may be creating some warmth in your heart down further down. Further and it intermingles with that red energy coming from the ground.

It's stabilized and gives you a spiritual link on the top of your head going up to infinity and grounding to the earth below. It makes you feel very healthy and very peaceful. This is the beginning of meditation-learning how to calm your body and you're relaxing. And to relax focus and being able to do other visualizations which will do things like bring energies into your body and open your chakras.

You can use this process to start practicing meditation on a regular basis. Just follow the relaxation technique for it to become second nature-and you can do different visualizations. When you're in a relaxed and centered mode. We're going to get ready to come out of this. What I want you to remember from this experience is the peace, the centeredness, and the focus of being in a relaxed but centered mode. This is the beginning of controlling your autonomic nervous system to doing this practice extensively over a period of time. It will help stabilize the autonomic nervous system and further stabilize your body.

A lot of visualizations you can do here will help that now. You'll be able to come down into this state and go even deeper when you practice these relaxation techniques. Let's start coming up. Nine- It is starting to get lighter and lighter as you are rising through the water-you're coming up. Eight-You start to see light-starting to be more aware of your surroundings. Seven coming out further-You feel light all around and you feel happy. You feel refreshed. Seven- coming out more you're in total consciousness. Six-higher up you feel filled with energy you feel relaxed-to feel healthy and feeling good. Five-surface-feeling good. Open your eyes slowly. So-this is the first exercise in meditation. Again you can use this exercise over and over to go to deeper states. Thank you for listening and I hope you enjoyed it.

Our Ego

(Transcription of Video)

Hello this is Marty Ettington. I'd like to tell you a story of the Ego. My story-I remember something that most people say you're not supposed to be able to. And how it gave me a greater understanding of the purpose of building an Ego. And how our search for spirituality transcends-so it goes back to a time before I was born. When I remember being part of a larger consciousness-and I was not on this Earth.

I felt that I was happy where I was. I also felt I had a mission that I had to accomplish back on Earth. Another consciousnesses was telling me that I didn't need to go back-that I had done enough. But I felt I needed to. So at some point I separated a small part of me from my consciousness and sent it back to earth to hunt for the proper parents. And I looked at several parents in upstate New York for the right set of qualities which I remember now was and I wanted. A set of parents that were very grounded in reality. It would help bring me up that way so I finally went close to one mother to be-who turned out to be my Mom. I got close to her and I was drawn inside into her womb and then I remember being in the womb. I remember from being very small-to growing and moving around and hearing sounds outside. My parents talking and the sounds around them. And then things seemed to be getting smaller inside there until my arms and legs were bumping up against the enclosure. At one point I remember the cord got around my neck and it was starting to choke me so I had to move to try and get into a better position and this ended up with my head away from the opening and my feet first out of the womb. So then things got smaller and smaller. I was growing, and growing, and finally I kicked and my mother's water broke. And everything contracted around me and then I remember being pulled out of the womb and it was so tight around my head. The pressure was unbelievable-it hurt horribly-then I was out.

And it was extremely cold outside. There were bright lights, and I was hit on the bottom-held up and hit on the bottom. I guess the doctor did it, and it hurt like hell. And I opened my mouth and cried and took my first breath of air which felt like fire. It was really painful but then the feeling went away quickly and I was breathing. But the doctor hit me again and I started to choke on some mucus and other things I guess. So they put me in an iron lung and I remember being in there and I know it was an hour or two and then things calmed down and I was breathing normally. So then I remember being taken home by my parents and the grandparents were all there and then I was passed around among them.

And I remember my grandmother on my father's side having bony arms and I didn't feel comfortable so I was crying. And then she said he doesn't like me and she passed me off to another one they said try again. And I understood what she was saying and I understood that I shouldn't cry to make her feel bad-so I didn't cry and she held me again, and it was OK.

Then I remember other instances of being in my crib, or my mom holding me close. My dad playing games with me. Anyway, unfortunately I got kind of thrown into the wall a little bit because he got too rambunctious-not on purpose. And I remember my entire babyhood. It's amazing learning to walk. When I was about two, I was sitting in front of a TV. And it's kind of when I woke up. It seemed that I'd been drifting for a couple years. I became aware of my surroundings and I said to myself-maybe not in these words-but saying "I'm here-I'm alive-I'm really here" so it was like a reality check. That I had been drifting through for the previous couple of years now.

I went through all the different things that growing up is about so anyway-Yes this is the best I remember. It really did happen to me. I don't know why I've never met anyone else who had a similar experience-but here's what I get from it. It is that when we're born we are a piece of pure spirit; we are a pure entity entering this world and the building of the Ego is a natural process.

It's how we deal with the environment around us because when we want something-especially as a baby we learn that by crying we will get attention. And as we get taken care of it feeds our sense of self-worth that the world responds to us-that all we need to do is to cry or make some other type of initiation of discomfort and people will take care of us. And as we get older we realize that's not going to work all the time and we become more integrated into our environment and the Ego acts is kind of a shell around our spirit. As we get older and live in civilization it's how we communicate with the environment. It shows we survived by having that Ego shell to keep us safe really.

And I believe that when we get to a certain point we can take one of two paths. We can either continue to focus on the Ego-the False Self and become more and more selfish- and lost in the Ego or we can be like a larva that's built a shell and is going to come out as a butterfly. By pursuing opportunities to reconnect with our spirit and by reconnecting with our spirit then we start by passing by the Ego. Here we start realizing the illusion of it; so it seems to me it's a natural growth path and that the Ego serves an important part in our being incarnated in this reality. That we can also transcend it and that's an important part of the reason for us to be here to be able to transcend it-to build that connection with our spirit. Thanks for listening to my story and I'll see you soon.

Enlightenment and Immortality

Enlightenment is a very popular subject as is Extended Longevity (Physical Immortality).

As spiritual beings we were put on this earth to develop our spirituality in a continuing evolution.

The spiritual development process also has the benefit of helping to increase our longevity.

Extended Longevity gives us needed time to continue to improve our connection to the Spiritual source in this life.

If we are not taking advantage of our God given abilities to improve our happiness and physical wellbeing then we are missing a significant potential in our lives.

The Author also reviews the extended longevity approaches he has learned and explained in his other books-along with some exercises to improve your overall health and longevity.

Introduction to Enlightenment & Immortality

There are thousands of books, lectures, ashrams, religions, and other approaches to developing spirituality.

All of these processes have value to the spiritual seeker.

There is also a high level of interest today in life extension through scientific, herbal, medical, spiritual, and even technological means.

Why the desire to live longer?

Could this be related to our search for meaning in life?

After having studied spiritual growth for much of my life, and extended longevity for the last several years, I have reached some conclusions on how the two subjects are not only related but critically interdependent on each other.

We generally need more time to develop our spiritual potential in this life, and so some of the basic reasons to desire extended longevity have to do with more potential for spiritual growth in the current incarnation.

My effort in this book is to tie spirituality and extended longevity together as the basis for a "Spiritual Longevity" set of life practices

Life is full of Pain and Suffering

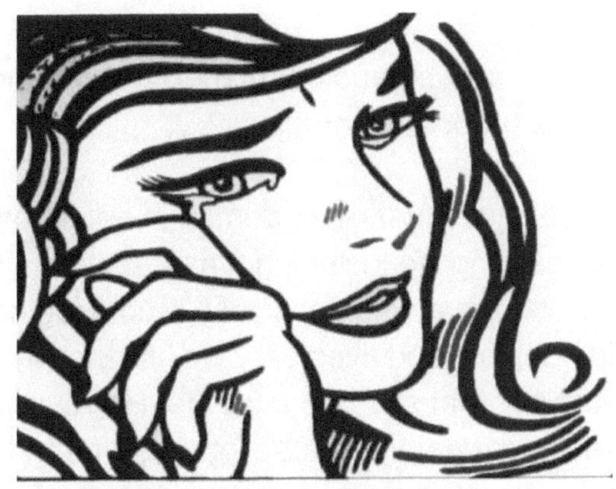

Do you ever wonder if life is worth living?

Are you retired and missing friends and family who have died before you?

Is there a reason to go on living?

Are you depressed because the life you had and people you used to know no longer exists or have died?

Do you wonder if there was ever an unfulfilled purpose missing in your life?

Would you like to live the years you have left in happiness and with purpose?

Is there a spiritual or God centered reason that our lives keep getting longer with each generation?

What is our purpose beyond career retirement and being grandparents?

How many of us as we get older start to wonder more and more about the purpose of our lives?

I recall a close family friend—a woman in her eighties; who had lived an exciting life including family, children, friends, and church. She traveled extensively, read a lot, had many friends and hobbies, and lived very well financially. Most people would say that she had a full life. However, one day she just got in her car in the closed garage, turned on the engine, and suffocated on purpose.

This woman lost her purpose in life and didn't take advantage of all the gifts she had to deepen her connection to God.

Life is full of suffering. In fact this truth was realized 2600 years ago in The Four Noble Truths by Gautama Buddha:

- *Life means suffering.*
- *The origin of suffering is attachment.*
- *The cessation of suffering is attainable.*
- *The path to the cessation of suffering.*

Being able to live in this world without letting the pain and suffering of life bother us is a worthy goal we can all strive for.

Isn't the pursuit of happiness written into the U.S. Declaration of Independence?

Our lives provide us the opportunity to learn how to reduce or eliminate our suffering and become one with God.

What Helps Us Handle Pain

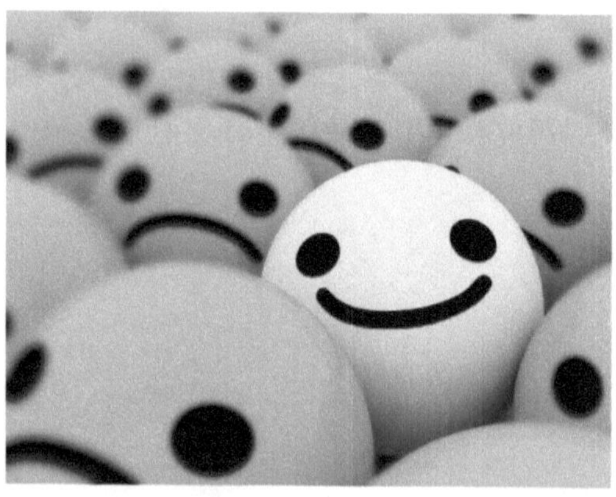

Spiritual growth helps our consciousness rise out of the earthy emotional and thought levels into more rapport with our own eternal spirit.

Anything that gets us to focus on something greater than ourselves will help us to avoid concentrating on the pain of our immediate existence.

Having a purpose and goals in life gives us reasons to live and something to look forward to in our lives.

Knowing that we can live a long healthy life also takes away many of the fears we have-especially when we are older and worried about how much real living we have left in our body.

Wouldn't it be great if we had much longer lives to work on our goals, dreams, and spiritual development to have a better chance of reaching our evolutionary potential?

Another factor to keep in mind is that we all have many illusions about reality and these illusions may be keeping us from becoming truly happy.

In my book "Removing Illusions to Find True Happiness" I discussed how illusions through our Ego affect our happiness:

When we are born we are pure and without an Ego.

I remember choosing my mother, being in here womb, and my birth. I did not have a focused central Ego when I was born—My being was just a core of pure spirit.
As we grow, the Ego starts to develop like a shell around our spirit. The Ego is what most of us think of as "I". It wants, it desires, it demands…..and when Ego doesn't get what it wants it becomes angry or depressed.

The Ego is a term commonly heard since it is used by psychologists a lot, but it is often misunderstood by most people.

The way psychologists use the word Ego may be different than it is often used in metaphysics and religious discussions and writings.

When I say Ego I mean an actual part of our energy body that builds an energy shell around our spirit. Most of our everyday experiences build this "shell" which becomes more solid and harder to crack or break as we become older.

Most of our culture focuses on the enhancement and satisfaction of this Ego shell.

The problem is that The Ego is not our true self but an illusion of our true self.

Therefore, the more we try to satisfy it the more we will become frustrated because the Ego can never be fully satisfied.

This is because the Ego is all about making you feel separate from other people and your surroundings.

Examples are how you feel "better than others", or "Smarter than others" or "Richer than others".

Much of what we do in life becomes an exercise in Ego because it often determines our self-worth such as:

- My girlfriend/boyfriend wants to be with me so I must be better than the other men available.

- Or—I just got a PHD in Physics from M.I.T. so I am smarter than a lot of other people and I will get to work on neat things that will be more fun and which will make me "happier" than I might otherwise be.

- I am in charge of a lot of people at work so I must be smarter and better than them.

The Ego is the basis of all illusions, and those illusions are also what cause misery in our lives.

The Ego In Our Lives

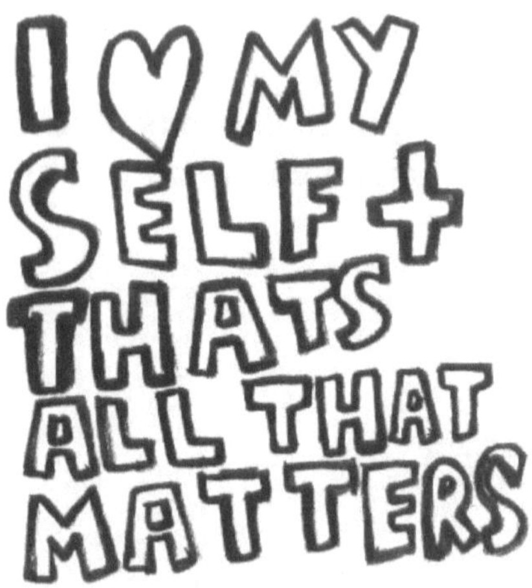

I was given a great gift before the beginning of my life, and I've only recently realized how great that gift was.

This gift was me being blessed with a continuous memory from before my conception--through birth—and until now.

I have clear experiences of remembering before my birth: Breaking off from a larger consciousness, choosing my mother, being in her womb, birth, and as a young baby.

Here is what I learned from remembering the incarnation and birth process….

The core of our being-our eternal spirit- tries to bring itself forward into our lives in each new incarnation.

We are all born with a piece of the spirit in us as the core of our consciousness.

As a newborn babe our minds are almost all made up of that spirit-and a sense of perception and curiosity about the world.

As the baby consciousness grows we learn about the world. While we do this we acquire an Ego. This Ego is part of our growth and helps us discern how to live in the world around us successfully.

It is a natural part of the growth of a baby to build this shell of thoughts and emotions around their spirit to become more aware of how to live in the world. Without this discernment we can't relate to our parents or our surroundings.

An analogy of this process might be that after shellfish drop older shells which are too small, they are very soft and vulnerable until their skin hardens into a new shell.

The building of our Ego shell is a similar protective mechanism.

The simple fact of learning to cry to get our mother's attention is how we learn to communicate to satisfy the needs of our bodies and to build the connection with our Mom and Dad; who help nurture us spiritually, emotionally, and physically.

I remember being hungry in my crib as a newborn baby and the only way I had to communicate was to cry—which babies do very effectively.

The usefulness of my crying was reinforced every time I did it—because I was hungry, had pooped or peed, or just wanted attention. Also, when I was hot, cold, or just unhappy.

This process steadily builds the infant ego as we all come to believe that our crying and desires control the universe around us.

As we become more aware and able to communicate, we start to understand that we are interacting with other beings—our parents and our family.

When I was about two years old I was sitting on the floor of my parent's living room watching cartoons on television. All of a sudden I felt like I had wakened from a dream. I saw everything around me much more clearly, and knew that I was alive and living in the world. It was my "I think therefore I am" moment.

I interpret this experience as being the moment my Ego congealed into a solid part of my consciousness. Everything going on around me became more understandable and clearer.

Parents naturally start to cut back on the total infant service as the child grows because they want the child to do age appropriate work for itself—feeding itself, using a toilet, getting dressed—all the steps a child goes through when they grow.

This process continues as we go to school and grow into adulthood.

Many people feel an emptiness as they grow and want to know more about themselves and why they are on this earth—they are searching for a connection to their eternal spirit.

Unfortunately, it's not so easy because the whole process of our growth into adults is normally in an environment which continues to value us as egocentric beings.

Take sports, grades, and all forms of competition. These are not bad—they are just part of everyday life and we are taught to make all of these activities and corresponding goals part of who we are.

This process naturally leads to us being centered in our artificial egos and we value the events and processes of the world as the main reality which we understand.

When we start exploring about who we really are, it is a learning process. Many of us turn to the religions in the cultures we are raised in.

Many of us have more of a passion and want to answer questions like:

- Why are we here?
- Who or what is God?

- Is my religion the best or only path to understanding?
- What is the meaning of life?

For most people with other priorities in life it may seem that we will never have time to explore the meaning of our lives and reach through our Ego to rebuild a deep connection with our spirit.

The growth of the Ego in each of us is a natural part of our lives on earth. However, we each have to make a conscious decision if we want to learn to feel the connection with our eternal spirit.

Longevity And Spirituality

I believe that our purpose in life is to experience this earth and evolve on it as spiritual beings.

A fortunate few learn how to feel the presence of the spirit in our everyday lives. Those persons become more and more enlightened as they build this connection with their spirit. It may be through learning prayer in a traditional religion like Christian Catholicism, or through meditation from the eastern philosophies and religious teachings.

Most people become caught in the everyday illusions of life and live with unhappiness in many forms due to their illusions.

This is where the expected roles of aging in a society create limitations.

The natural sequence in all societies is to be born, grow into adulthood, work, marry, have children, raise the children, retire, live a few years, and then die.

It seems a terrible tragedy that most of the people ever born on this earth are so caught up in the travails of everyday life that they never get beyond the packaged beliefs they are raised in to see the truth of their spirit for themselves.

Most people's free time for self-examination is very limited due to the daily activities of their lives—even into old age. We are talking about 99% of the population.

What can be done about this problem? How are we to help the masses have the opportunity for spiritual growth and self-fulfillment into becoming more realized beings?

After much thought and meditation I've concluded that helping each of us to have the potential for much longer lives than is now common would help us address what I would like to call the "life gap of enlightenment".

In my separate research and writings I've documented many persons who have lived well over the age of 150 years—some into the several hundred year range.

I now believe that my interest in the subject some years ago was driven by a subconscious spiritual knowledge of the importance extended longevity to create more opportunities for our spiritual growth.

Think about it—adding many more years beyond the normal lifetime naturally provides a greater opportunity for an individual's introspection and growth.

Once a person reaches the age of a "Senior" (commonly starting the in the fifties and beyond), they have experienced most of what normal life has to offer—love, careers, family, death of those close to you, accomplishment, and the seeing the results of their efforts here on earth. What is left?

The older one gets, the more they have "boredom" with the world and want to learn about their reason for being. This curiosity may come out of hiding in their subconscious after a lifetime of being suppressed below the other priorities of living in the world day to day.

Providing more time for a person to search for the truth in their lives thus allows them to have a greater chance to reach a greater enlightenment about themselves and a greater connection with their spirit.

It's also interesting to note that when studying the lives and teachings of very old persons—these people know that one of the main components of extreme longevity is being centered in the spirit.

I use as an example the well documented case of Li-Ching-Yung who lived to 256 years and who said his secret to a long life was:

 "Keep Quiet heart, Sit Like a Tortoise, Sleep Like a Dog"

A "quiet heart" in the speech of the east refers to being in touch with your core being or spirit. Sitting like a tortoise also has to do with living in a slower and more thoughtful way.

So we can see that living with a closer connection to our spirit is not only a way to reach a more enlightened and happier state within us, but the action of doing that brings that spirit down into our bodies to increase our overall health and longevity.

Now we have a connection between extended longevity and the spiritual value of that additional lifespan.

One could say that the search for the spiritual connection in our lives also has a byproduct of extending our lives.

To what end do we want to do this? My intuition tells me that the purpose is to allow many more of us to become realized beings in this life.

Isn't that what the cycle of birth and death is all about? To become a further evolved and realized being at the end?

To become more spiritually evolved is to become more enlightened. What is enlightenment? Do we understand what the state is that we are striving to reach?

More About Enlightenment

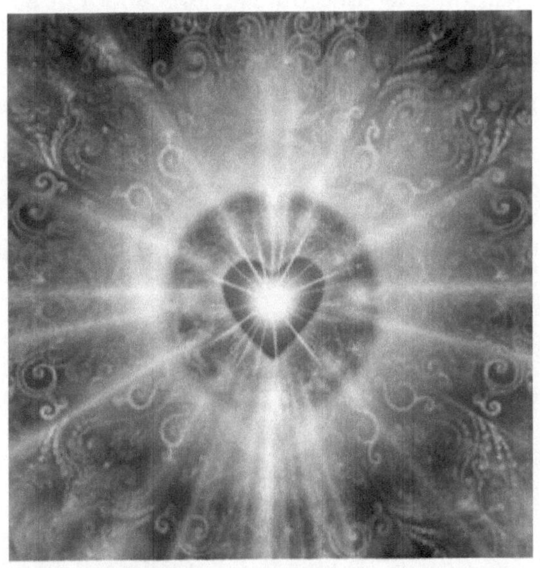

Enlightenment is a state that is impossible to understand unless you actually reach it.

Enlightenment is like a man who can see brilliant color in the land of the blind who only understand black and white.

<u>How is this state related to longevity and Immortality?</u>

- The more Enlightened you are, the easier it is to synchronize your Spirit, Energy, and Physical bodies (which we will discuss more later in this book)

- Enlightenment helps you to pierce the illusions most of us live under about ourselves and our environment—and our illusions about death

- Happiness allows you to have more positive outlook on life and to visualize positively about your health and future

- Many immortals are enlightened, and the same is true of enlightened masters—most are as immortal as they choose to become

- The two concepts are directly related and balance each other

  - An immortal has much more time to perfect their enlightenment

  - An enlightened person has a much easier time perfecting their body to be immortal

<u>What is Enlightenment?</u>

Start by looking at what Enlightenment is not:

- Enlightenment is not getting something whether that's getting more knowledge or becoming spiritually advanced.

- We need to let go of what we think it means to be spiritual

- Enlightenment has nothing to do with living up to a spiritual ideals

- We need to let go of any preconceived ideas about what meditation practice is and what it will do for you.

One of my favorite sayings on enlightenment is from Andrew Cohen's book "Enlightenment is a Secret"

On Page 60: *"Spiritual is the very nature of what you already are. There is nothing to do about it except to realize it. Once you have made this discovery it's all over."*

- Enlightenment is the continuous state of knowing that you are the source energy at all times in every moment of life.

- Enlightenment is something you are, not something you go and get. This is why enlightenment does not need to be sought.

Enlightenment cannot be discerned by reading about it, it can only be experienced
(Be Here Now-Baba Ram Dass)

First a foremost you must understand that you are a Spiritual being having a human experience.

You are the energy you a looking for.

Right here. Right NOW.

This practice is simply an exploration of what is already present in you.

Enlightenment is a certainty that never leaves you. (Master Nasargadata)

It is a certainty that is so profound it can be called "remembering," because the truth of your being is so constant it becomes impossible to forget.

Certainty is more than the lack of doubt, fear and indecision.

Certainty is accompanied by trust.

When I look inside and see that I am nothing, that is wisdom, when I look outside, and see that I am everything, That's LOVE, and between these two my life turns.

Examples of the State of Enlightenment:

"Be Here Now" By Baba Ram Dass—Living in the Now

Feeling the Oneness of everyone and everything around you which is a state of boundless love

(Imagine feeling towards everyone and everything the way you feel about the person you love most in life)

<u>Enlightenment in Opening the Heart</u>

The gradual unfolding of our spirit within our bodies involves the opening of different chakras including the heart chakra.

The heart chakra is the center of love in our bodies and thus is our strongest connection to the spirit of God we can feel.

While I learned to open my crown chakra to take in vital forces energy and have a better connection to the divine at a young age, I didn't know what I was missing in my heart until very recently.

Learning exercises to open the heart chakra a couple of years ago gave me some very powerful but limited experiences with experiencing the energy of an unconditional love of God force within me.

This state is where you start to radiate Love to all of those around you and it fills your heart with happiness as you connect more broadly throughout your body and to others.

Recently my heart chakra opened completely on a daily basis and its (Ettington M. K., Love From The Heart, 2012) effect on me has been profound.

I love to sit for hours and just enjoy the heat and joy within my chest and my connection to everyone-it is like a drugged natural high.

I see all of my friends in a new light. This experience makes me realize that for most of my life I had a deep gap and loneliness in my heart which has only now been filled after living fifty plus years in this life. I had thought that intimacy with woman could fill that hole within me. That is not how it works.

Now, I realize the fallacy of that belief. We can really only fill loneliness with a connection to the spirit of God through our hearts.

This love from God is something I want to share with everyone and help everyone learn to open their hearts too.

<u>The Limits of Enlightenment</u>

Unlike many other seekers I believe that enlightenment is a continuous process—not a single blaze of light and understanding.

We live in an infinite Universe and there are beings of much greater power and glory than we can conceive.

Every time we reach a new state of enlightenment we find that the road ahead is still infinitely long and forever full of wonderful mysteries.

Why not take advantage of living our lives as fully and as long as possible to evolve to our full potentials?

Why are We Alive?

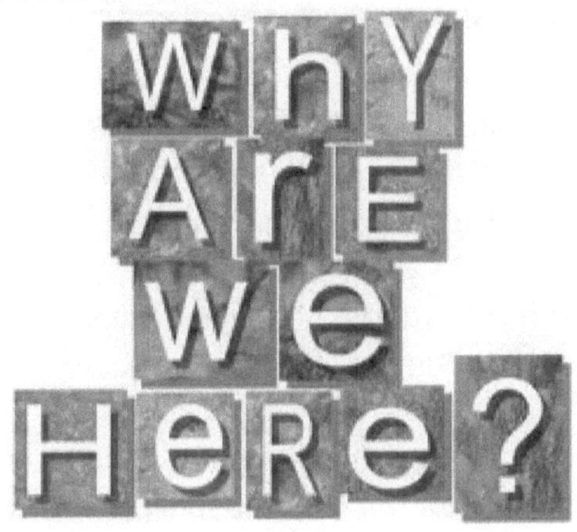

What do most of us do with our lives? We live it day to day-and don't usually give much thought to why we are here.

Most of us do not have a choice--we have to go to school, to work, to take care of a family--for most of our lives.

Even in economically advanced countries we only have a few years left at the end of our lives to spend much time thinking our ultimate purpose on earth.

Why so short a time?

What if we could have many more years of living?

Why would we want to do with extra time?

Deciding what to do with our lives is a decision only we can make—because each of us only knows our own heart.

A quote on the meaning of life:

"Life has no meaning. Each of us has meaning and we bring it to life. It is a waste to be asking the question when you are the answer." — Joseph Campbell

The above is a great quote because it talks about the meaning we each bring to life.

Since my experiences tell me that we all come back and incarnate on earth for our own reasons, we do all bring meaning to each of our lives.

It is up to each of us to work out that meaning in each of our lives.

The time we have on earth is to allow us to work out issues which will help perfect our beings.

It may also be to resolve old issues from previous incarnations.

However much time we have on this earth it always seems too short. This is why it takes so many lifetimes to work out our "Karma".

What if we could extend our life much longer than currently possible? Wouldn't this give us the time we need to resolve the issues in our beings which were our goals for our current life on this Earth?

But first we would need a deep purpose in living—
otherwise why bother.

*Without a well-developed purpose in life we have no
reason to make the effort to grow spiritually towards
becoming perfected beings.*

The Importance of Extended Longevity

For a few people, spiritual awakenings come early in life because of positive karma, or through a spontaneous experience. However, most of us have to work at it for many years to make breakthroughs.

Even though I have been a spiritual seeker most of my life, my awakenings have been gradual over a long period of time; and are still going on.

In the nineteen sixties when I was a boy there wasn't much aside from the Bible at our house in small town in upstate New York as a guide for the spiritual path. Don't get me wrong-the Bible is a great document of History, Religion, and Spirituality—but there is much more to learn in other texts and experiences about spiritual paths.

I did read a book called "Stranger Than Science" By Frank Edwards which had a series of unbelievable and supposedly true stories which posed some major questions to me that nobody I knew could answer.

At the RPI where I was studying engineering in the early seventies I found a mentor—a physics graduate student in his forties named Sam-who was also an accomplished clairvoyant and healer.

Sam introduced me to meditation and the opening of my crown chakra. This was a major milestone in my life and the results were incredible.

As my vital forces increased and I opened up spiritually and psychically.

I had experiences of prophecy, astral projection, learned to do healing, and many other awakenings. I was only nineteen years old.

For the next several decades my career, family, and the routines of daily life became my priorities and although I meditated and continued to read a lot I felt stuck –that I was not spiritually advancing.

My next milestone was aided with technology- when I bought a new type of Meditation CD (from Centerpointe) which played two different frequency tones in my ears and turned my haphazard meditations into consistently deep and steady ones.

Over a period of eight of nine years, I continued to become calmer and more centered. That period was also when I had many prophecies about major events and my life.

(Profiled in my book Prophecy: A History and How to Guide)

Then I seemed to plateau again for several years….

My divorce started in 2008 and this led me to write my well known book on Immortality: "Physical Immortality: A History and How to Guide"

The other effect of my divorce was to lead me to re-evaluate my life—my goals, my social life, and what I wanted to do for the rest of my life.

I took up new practices including learning Reiki Healing—where I went to numerous classes and took several levels of training and certification.

This process included more exercises to open chakras and manipulate vital forces.

Then I learned a exercise to open the heart chakra which resulted in a couple of amazing experiences of powerful unconditional love.—which each lasted a few hours then want away again.

Two years and many spiritual groups and classes later my heart chakra opened fully and brought me to a whole new level of awareness.

My heart opening has become a great blessing in my life and is even more powerful than my crown chakra opening several decades ago.

To feel the love of God in my heart fills a hole that I know now I've had my whole life—and I didn't even realize how empty my heart was.

To feel filled with love and this life force pulsing throughout my chest is a wonderful experience.

It is hard to explain the joy of feeling a connection of love to everyone and everything around one-but it is worth it.

I know now that as my life goes on I will continue to develop spiritually and will have many more wonderful experiences.

So far my spiritual journey has been about forty-five years, and I'm still having major experiences as time goes on.

These continued experiences give me a strong desire to want to stay on this earth as long as I can-to build an ever deeper connection to my spirit.

I'm just getting to what most people would call "Senior" adult status, but my spiritual growth is constantly renewing itself and will continue to do so for many more years.

Having another couple of centuries or more in my life will not be enough time to explore and experience everything I want to in this varied and beautiful world we live on.

Extended Longevity provides the additional time most of us need to learn and experience meaning and spiritual growth in our lives.

How do we Lengthen our Lives?

In addition to taking advantage of modern medical science, nutrition, and exercise, there is a spiritual and holistic approach to extended longevity and long term health.

One of my beliefs from the evidence I've studied is that the Ego creates a barrier to long term health.

The reason is that the Ego interferes with the ability of the spirit to come down into our physical bodies.

Why is that? It's because our bodies were designed to operate with a pure controlling influence of the spirit affecting our energy fields, which affect our physical bodies.

When our thoughts and emotions which build our Ego are stressed, or negative, or limiting then this eventually affects our incarnations in a physical way.

This lack of connection between our spirit and our physical bodies is also reflected in the actions of vital forces in our energy bodies. These channels can become clogged-another reason the body can get sick.

A Spiritual Holistic Approach to Health then should consist of the following steps and focuses for action:

- Building a soul based statement of purpose and goals for your life. This can be done at any age, but reviewing the life purpose when a person is in middle age or older will help to refocus your soul purpose.

- Changing the "Psychology of Death" to the "Psychology of Living". A person has to know in their heart that their lifespan can be much longer than they were taught by society what is possible. Once the individual has the purpose to live longer, and the solid confidence and belief that they can live longer, they are ready to take charge of their own paths.

- Spiritual work in terms of meditation, visualization, and other exercises of the mind and spirit to let them open themselves to God or higher consciousness.

- Energy work from different practices to do energy work on the body to help their energies flow and revitalize their life forces. These practices can include anything from Tai Chi, to Qi Gong, to Kundalini raising practices.

- Enhancing the physical body. In addition to the normal good health and diet practices we can learn, we should also take some longevity herbal supplements to help our bodies stay young and fit.

- Learning to use our spirit to see and avoid danger in our future. You're your body is healthy the biggest danger to longevity becomes accidents. Various techniques help us learn how to improve our safety on a daily basis—since none of us wants to die by accidents do we?

There are a variety simple techniques and approaches we can use to extend our longevity for many years— but we have to have an open mind first.

Synchronization of Spirit, Energy, Physical Body

You are not just your physical body. Your being includes a Spiritual Core, an Energy Body, and Physical Body.

These are concepts which are woven into many religions and philosophies, with related energy body concepts mostly being understood in the East more than the West.

Many believe that your entire being consists of at least three states as described below.

The Spirit

Here we mean the spirit which is your "soul" or core of your being. An individual's spirit is one with the God spirit and is present in every person and every being. It exists outside of time and space. This is a place some call "no time and no space". It is everywhere present simultaneously.

The spirit exists in all things and each person has that same core spirit within them.

We can learn to live focused more in the spirit through a variety of religious, meditational, and philosophical traditions.

The Energy Body

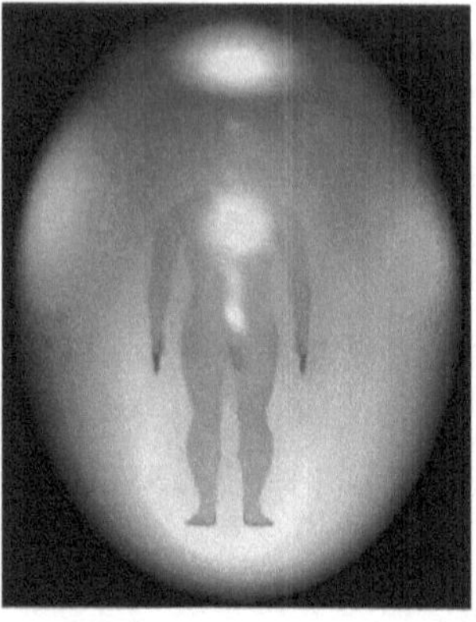

Some organizations like the Hindus and Theosophists believe we have multiple energy body levels. The Theosophists believe there are at least six distinct energy bodies.

Many other traditions only talk about one energy body which provides the life force to energize our physical bodies.

The acupuncture meridians and chakras are all parts of the energy body which exists in very close proximity to the physical body.

The aura is also a manifestation of the energy body too, which overlaps your physical body.

Many people claim to be able to see "auras" including this Author. The aura is the physical energy manifestation of the energy body. All living people have an aura and one can tell a lot about their health by how their aura looks.

The Physical Body

This is the body most of us know, and that most of us think is all of us that exists. This is the body we want to heal and energize to achieve physical immortality.

Exercises done on the physical body also affect the energy body.

Herbal supplements work from the physical body to help correct energy flows in your energy body.

How the Bodies Work Together

Spiritual development exercises and physical exercises help increase the synchronization of these bodies.

By bringing the absolute peace and stillness of the spirit down into the energy and physical bodies you increase the perfection and health of those bodies.

This is since in the normal course of events the stresses of our life cause more randomness or entropy in our energy and physical bodies. These stresses of daily life age us prematurely and cause disease.

We can repair our energy and physical bodies by integrating them better with the spiritual body; and getting the energies to flow in the correct patterns, chakras, and meridians, and with more vital force.

The specific practices to extend your longevity are provided in much more detail in "Physical Immortality: A History and How to Guide".

Synchronization is a holistic approach of working on our entire being to help us become healthier, happier, and to have much more profound life experiences.

Connecting to the Spirit

The Importance of Stillness

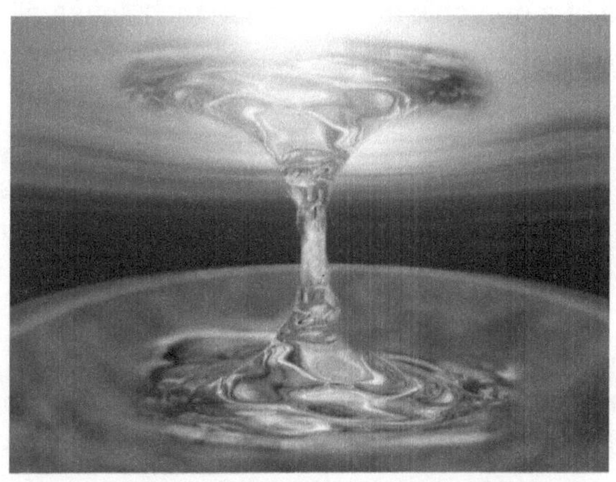

How does spiritual growth help one stay healthy; and what is stillness?

The ideas I'm going to discuss here relate to eastern Asian concepts of the spirit as taught mainly in China and India.

Buddhism, Taoism, Zen, and other eastern religions and philosophies all teach that the spirit is the core of our being; and that our physical bodies are just an extension of that spirit into the physical level of existence.

By learning to let your mind or ego release its hold on the illusion of our current existence, we become aware of the spirit behind or at the core of our being. This spirit is the pure oneness of God and exists in no time and no space.

(A concept which we really can't envision with our minds or egos only).

There are many techniques taught to get closer to realizing the core of a person's being. These techniques all involve practicing spiritual growth, love, and/or meditation with a goal of enlightenment.

There are thousands of books and practices on this subject so I will not try to duplicate them in this short synopsis.

The Chinese stress that the stillness and oneness obtained through spiritual growth are one of the main keys to keeping the body healthy for a long life. Many Taoist techniques and teachings stress the achievement of "stillness" as a prelude to physical immortality.

The stillness I'm referring to is found mainly through meditation. In Christian terms it is often referred to as the "Peace that passes all understanding".

It is hard to describe the feeling of stillness since it is like when you first wake up in the morning after a deep sleep—but even quieter and deeper.

The feeling of stillness has a strong effect on your body—it seems to make the randomness of your cells quiet down into a more restful state.

Meditation is taught many places; I've even found a company which sells CDs that help even beginners achieve deep states of relaxation that usually takes advanced Yogis years of practice.

Stillness is not something achieved overnight but takes years, (even with modern advanced CD techniques) to start showing results.

However, the effects of stillness practices probably have the most profound effects on your body's aging as anything else I can recommend.

This is since as you start to achieve stillness, your Ego is realizing its core is really part of the spirit—not a separate mind. The spirit exists outside time and space. This connection with your spirit has a profound health effect on the body in terms of peace and well-being.

When meditating in this state you can feel stillness penetrating your body.
It feels like your body is reaching a relaxed state never realized; even in sleep.
The state of the stillness of your spirit provides a modified blueprint for your body's health.

It is a lot of work to set aside time every day to meditate. The good news is you will find that after some weeks of practicing, this time becomes something you look forward to. This is since meditation is so relaxing it becomes a way to recharge you for daily activities in the world.

I also find that meditation makes my mind more alert when I wake up in the morning and gives me a sharper intellectual edge at work.

The Reality of Stillness

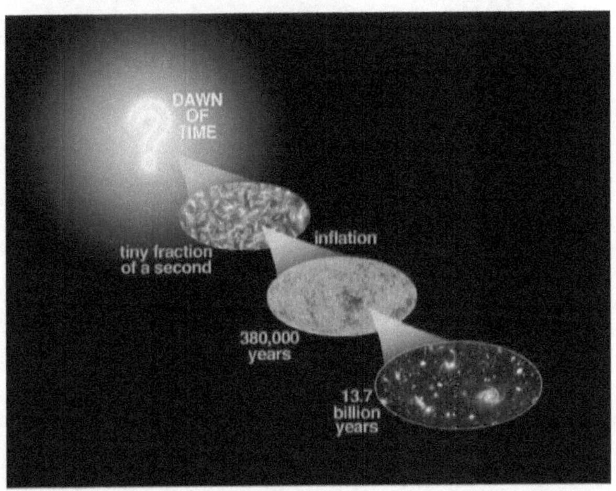

Most people believe that God was the initial creative force which started the Universe.

Physicists and Astronomers all agree that the Universe we know was created from nothing and inflated in a huge explosion called the "Big Bang". As it inflated time and space as we know them came into existence.

When you study Einstein's Relativistic physics you being to understand that time and space are inextricably linked. You can't have one without the other.

Given our understanding of physics, we know that time and space didn't exist before the Big Bang. The state of things before creation was "No Time & No Space".

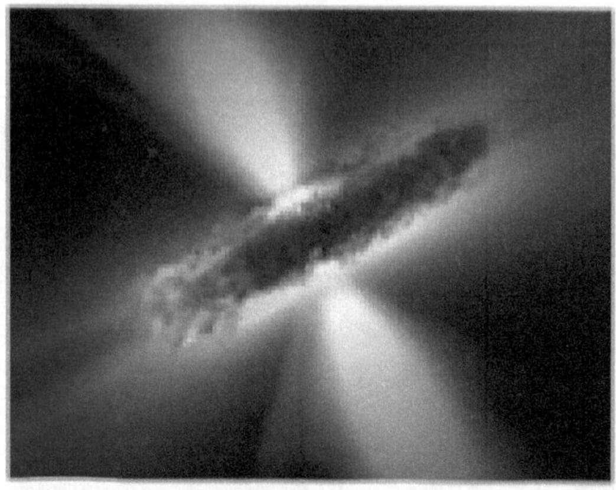

Another subject of great interest to astrophysicists is what are called "Black Holes". Black Holes are a result of Einstein's equations and astronomers have verified their existence in the last few decades.

Black Holes are stars which due to their own mass have collapsed down to an infinitely small point where time stops. Scientists do not understand where all that mass goes.

Hmm.... A   Black Hole seems to be another example of part of reality that exists without time and space.

In Quantum Physics, time is also viewed differently than we perceive it on a daily basis. Here is a quote from a Physics website explaining this view:

> *The upshot is that, on the microscopic level, there is no direction to time -- and this is even more spectacularly true in quantum physics than in*

> *classical physics. In the microscopic domain, everything just exists in a kind of nebulous, atemporal continuum. Then, every once in a while, something becomes observable, and enters the one-dimensional time continuum. The arrow of time does not exist in the universe as a whole. It only exists in individual subjective views of the universe!*

I think it is fair to say that the place of stillness where time and space don't exist is part of our reality.

Therefore, it shouldn't be considered too strange that our immortal spirit is part of and one with that stillness.

Finding Stillness in Major Religions

Christianity is the largest religion in the world, and one I know pretty well since I was raised in Methodist and Presbyterian churches growing up. I also attended multiple churches as an adult and participated in Bible study groups for a number of years.

Prayer is the key to stillness as a Christian. There are many books on Prayer and Prayer techniques. One needs to focus on spirit and becoming one with the spirit to move towards a state of stillness as a Christian.

The fact that so many of the long lived persons recorded in this book lived in Christian cultures probably indicates that being a devoted Christian can help you "live in the spirit" as much as many other spiritual techniques.

I'm not as familiar with Judaism and Islam, but the same approach applies in doing prayers in those religions.

The key to Prayer in your religion or spiritual approach is that you must learn to focus on the spirit of God which is inside you; and is the core of your being. That spirit exists in eternal peace; outside of time and space.

Once you learn to focus on that spirit in your prayer you will be able to bring that peace and stillness into your physical body to calm it and provide more health.

<u>Biblical Quotes Relating to Stillness and the Spirit</u>

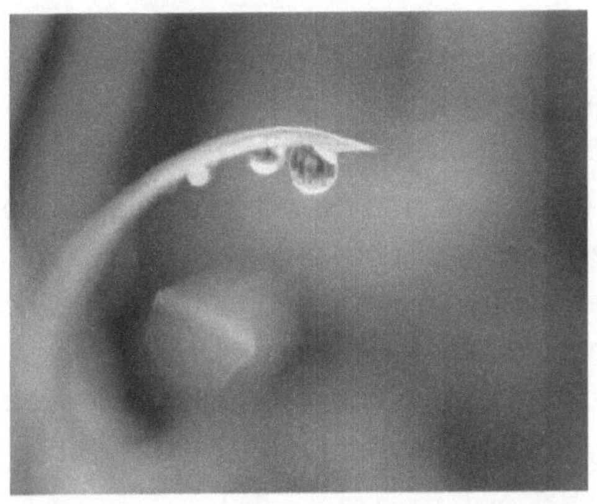

Here are a number of Biblical quotes which relate to the power of the spirit and the state of stillness (peace) I've described above.

You will experience God's peace which is far more wonderful than the human mind can understand. His peace will keep your thoughts and your hearts quiet and at rest as you trust in Jesus Christ. (Philippians 4:7 LB)

He will keep in perfect peace all those who trust in him, whose thoughts turn often to the Lord. (Isaiah 26:3 LB)

The work of righteousness shall be peace; and the effect of righteousness, quietness and assurance forever. (Isaiah 32:17 KJV)

"You shall receive power when the Holy Spirit has come upon you; and you shall be my witnesses both in

Jerusalem, and in all Judea and Samaria,   and even to the remotest part of the Earth. (Acts 1:8 NASB)

For by one Spirit are we all baptized into one body (1 Corinthians 12:13 KJV)

I will ask the Father and he will give you another Comforter, and he will never leave you. He is the Holy Spirit. The spirit who leads into all truth. The world at large cannot receive him; for it isn't looking for him and doesn't recognize him. But you do, for he lives with you now, and some day shall be in you. (John 14:16,17 LB)

Do you not know that you are a temple of God and that the spirit of God dwells within you? (1 Corinthians 3:16 NASB)

There are many more quotes about the spirit of God, but the key is that they all relate to that core of God's spirit inside us all.

The search for stillness is the search for God within us. Stillness makes its presence felt within our physical body as well as in our spirit.

Energy Flows and Chakra Development

There are many traditions of vital forces development for the human body. In this Chapter we will just cover some basic concepts and a simple exercise.

The Chinese concept of energy meridians (the points and channels along which energy moves) are used in acupuncture therapy and are another way of looking at the energy flows a body needs.

These and the Indian concept of energy centers (chakras) are all about the way your energy body is designed to stay healthy when energy flows are working properly.

Below is a diagram of the main acupuncture meridians of the body:

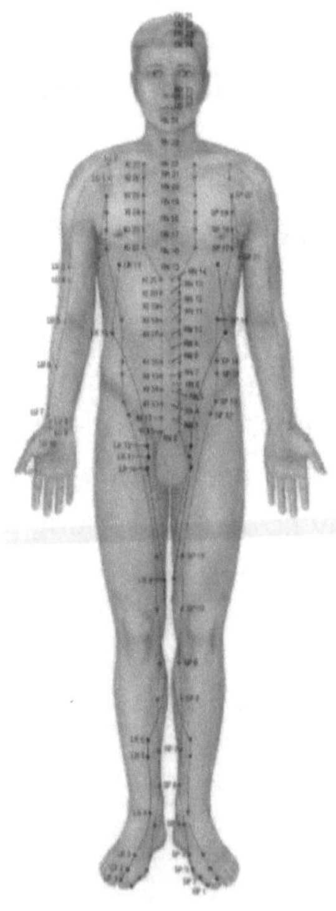

When those flows are interrupted it affects our health and acupuncture can be used to restore this. Needles are used by acupuncturists to stop and start energy moving at key meridian points to help restore the energy body to a proper balance.

Chakra development exercises also help repair energy flows.

In many persons the energy is often not flowing properly
and has to be repaired.
These improvements help one's health; and as the energy
starts moving properly again.

As a result the energy body starts affecting the physical
body in a more healthy way.

Many books and traditions discuss details of energy
meridians and chakra development so I will not do so here.
A short summary of Chakras and their functions follows.

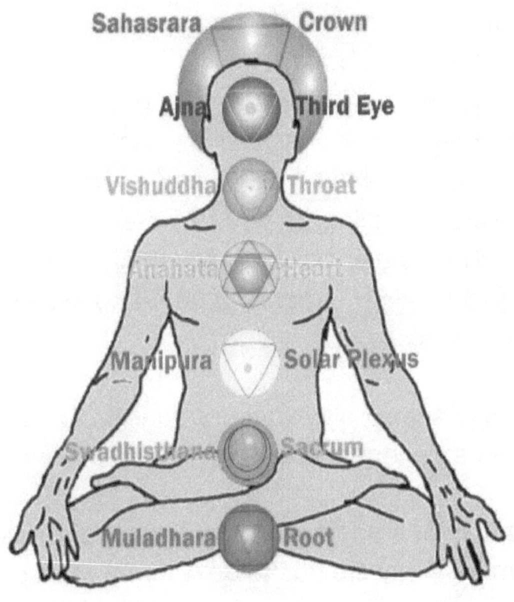

The Figure above shows the chakra centers on the body.
These chakras are energy centers where you take in
energy to keep your body healthy. The chakras when

developed are commonly thought to control spiritual and mental abilities as follows:

- <u>Crown Chakra</u>: *To be open, to know, intuition, precognition, connection   with infinite intelligence, to have faith and connection with God*
- <u>3rd eye Chakra</u>: *Clairvoyance, psychic reading, to have vision or insight, photographic memory and telekinesis*
- <u>Throat Chakra</u>: *Communication center, telepathy, clairaudience, inner   voice and tone healing*
- <u>Heart Chakra</u>: *To be in affinity with, to be at one with, to connect with, compassion and unconditional love*
- <u>Solar Plexus Chakra</u>: *Astral projection, to be empowered, to manifest, to   be in control of yourself, psychic healing and levitation*
- <u>Sacrum/Feeling Chakra</u>: *Clairsentience, emotional feelings, balance of   male and female energies*
- <u>Root Chakra</u>: *Grounding, realizing, letting go, and surviving*

Meditation is almost always a prerequisite to being able to develop these energy centers.

One example of a positive youthful effect of Chakra development in my life has to do with my head of hair.

I've been developing my crown chakra since I was 18 years old. Now in my fifties, all the men in my family are well on the way to being bald at my age.

However, I still have a full head of hair. I attribute this to the energies which come into my crown chakra daily and which have extended the life of my hair follicles.

The root chakra is where the Kundalini comes from. One must be careful in developing this one since it can cause major imbalances in the others.

It is recommended to find a worthy instructor to develop these energy centers as part of a spiritual development process.

Below is a Crown Chakra Energy Intake Exercise which works well for me.

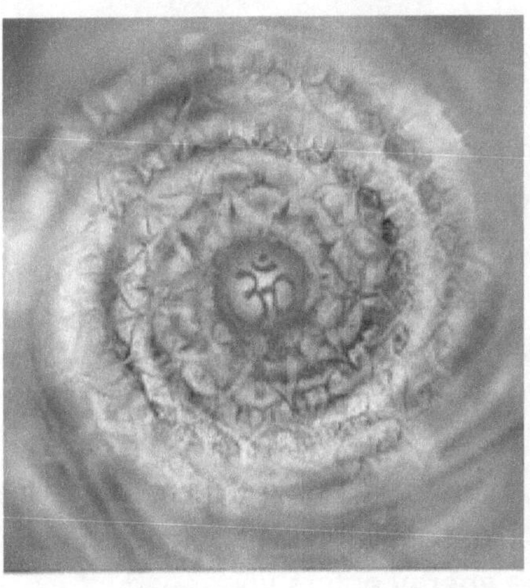

The following exercise on taking in energy through your crown chakra works very well for me and helps energize the energy pathways and chakras in my body. I've used this approach successfully for years.

It may take several times doing this before you start to feel the heat in the top of your head as a result.

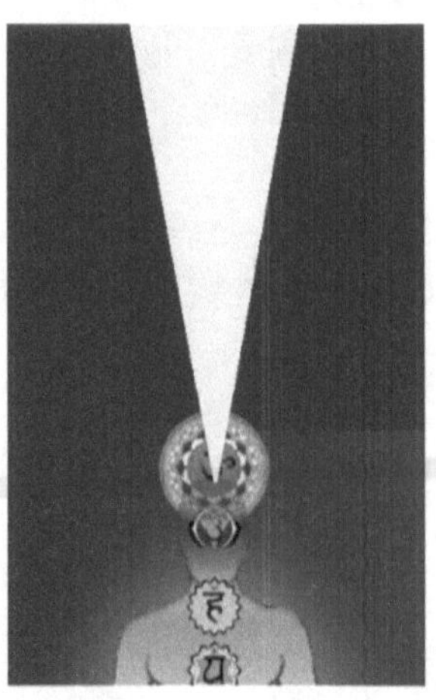

- Go through a 5-10 minute relaxation exercise while sitting up.

- Now visualize a large cone coming from infinity into the top of your head. (See above) It intersects the crown chakra.

- Also, visualize your crown chakra as the 1000 petal lotus blossom which is opening as you will it; and as the energy enters your head.

- Imagine a large amount of energy and white light is funneling down   towards your head, and that as it does so the energy becomes more compressed and more powerful.

- The energy enters your head and when it starts to flow you should feel heat in the top of your head; then the energy will flow into your body.

- Keep using your will to pump in the energy. First send it to open your third eye to take in energy there too.

- Now the energy travels down your neck to open the throat chakra.

- Next the energy pours into your chest. When it really gets going it's like a pleasant warmth or fire in your chest. Keep visualizing the energy condensing into the funnel and going into your head and down your body as we continue this exercise.

- Next the energy opens your heart and solar plexus chakras. As those open you will feel more energy pouring into your chest; and in the case of the heart chakra—unconditional love.

- As the energy travels down your chest it reaches your navel and your sacrum chakra. As it reaches that chakra, again feel it opening and energy pouring into you.

- At last the energy reaches your root chakra at the base of the spine. The   root chakra also draws fiery energy from beneath the earth. This energy is called Kundalini.

- Now imagine that your root chakra is anchored into the ground; and this Kundalini fire will pass upwards through your spine. You feel the fire coursing up your spine and eventually into your head.

- Now you have the full flow of energies throughout the major chakras of your body. Keep visualizing the energy coming in through your crown and circulating down to the root; and then the Kundalini circling back up. As this happens it opens all your energy centers more and you will feel the energy pouring into you. (Do this for five more minutes)

Our energy body has many pathways and energy centers. Keeping those paths open and energy centers functioning is a key component to our spiritual and physical health.

Summary of Enlightenment and Immortality

We are all beings with a core of eternal spirit that all have free will.

Our civilization and knowledge is now at a point where we can decide how long we want to live on this earth.

We are continuously evolving not only individually but as a race of beings. I believe it is our destiny to eventually evolve into powerful spiritual beings that will be to us as we are to one celled life.

Our higher consciousness put us here on this earth to work on our spiritual growth.

Instead of just drifting through life without a purpose, we can have full meaning in our lives not just daily, but minute to minute, second to second.

This means developing a life purpose and goals. We can do this at any age.

We can make a conscious decision as to how much time we want to live in this life to reach our life's purpose and goals.

After we have established our "Soul's Purpose" then we can learn practices and techniques to extend our lives much longer than we thought was possible.

Summary

In this course we spent a lot of time on your Spiritual Connection. No matter what religion or belief system you have, it's important to have some type of connection to God.

This connection is really to your inner spirit which lives outside of time and space.

There are various ways to connect to your spirit through prayer, meditation, and communing with nature. What is important is that you do something.

This connection is the most important thing you can do to build your long term health and happiness.